# Hijama vs. Cupping

## No Ijaaza, No Hijama

Understanding and Protecting the Ancient Art of Hijama Therapy

**James M. McConnell**

Broken Earth Publishing Inc.
Independence, VA
USA

**First Edition**

**Rabi Al-Awwal 1434 / January 2013**

**Printed in the USA**



ISBN 978-1-62507-002-9

# Disclaimer

The author of this book is not a medical doctor licensed by any state and does not intend to make any claims of a medical nature. No opinions set forth in these pages have been evaluated by the United States FDA.

Hijama as described in this book is a "healing art" falling under the definition of a religious practice, more specifically, a practice performed by Prophet Muhammad (saws). It is his example that is being described herein and any benefits obtained both physical and spiritual through the practice of the Sunnah of Hijama are gifts from the Creator for maintaining good health.

This book is for informational purposes and is not intended to qualify the reader to perform hijama.

Qualification can only come from an authorized teacher with an ijaaza and through direct authorized teaching and practice.

# Introduction

Known by many names, practiced by many cultures, hijama (fire/wet cupping) is a practice that has quickly gained much attention in the West. The danger arises when capitalistic influences, driven by the profit motivated medical industry; encroach on ancient, conservative, proven, holistic and religious treatments that were entrusted to healers, not businessmen. We are now in an age controlled by the medical mafia. No matter if treatments are termed conventional or alternative, buyer beware.

A few years ago there were only a couple of places to learn about hijama (really cupping) and have it performed. Since then a number of websites and unauthorized practitioners have entered the fold and, as alluded to on our website when first launched, they are influenced by economic concerns, their own egos, prestige, ignoring our many warnings. Many people have taken what we have offered, reworked it, directly lifted information, added some fantastic and unsupported medical claims and are currently setting up their own industry without ever having an ijaaza to practice this ancient and extremely important sunnah. All clear indicators on how critically important having an ijaaza is to practice hijama. In the end, those who enter this field to inflate their own ego and support their pockets will unfortunately find themselves bankrupt on the Day of Judgment. May Allah (swt) save us from such false prophets, scholars and practitioners, and send us a true leader (Sultan) who can revive the glory of Islam.

Hijama is a practice governed by the superior and advanced

Ijaaza based system of education.

**Anyone practicing hijama without an Ijaaza is not practicing hijama, they are practicing cupping.**

Despite the pages filled with quotes or hadith from our beloved Prophet (saw), authorization to practice hijama can only come with ijaaza, not self promotion, high claims, advanced marketing techniques, and fancy language. Without an ijaaza to perform Hijama the spiritual component is missing and without the spirit (God connection), there is no hijama. This is the primary distinction between hijama and cupping. Hijama is rooted in a God-fearing morally grounded system of health and belief as prescribed by Prophets and Saints connected to the Creator of all things. No connection, no hijama. Hijama is a spiritually based practice following the Sunnah of Prophet Muhammad (saw) therefore it is a religious practice, not a medical procedure.

We would strongly urge people seeking the many benefits of hijama to avoid these false teachers and practitioners and in doing so help preserve the integrity and high stations that are associated with true healing practices. People are free to do as they like, we are not here to police people. We only want to fulfill our duty to warn those who might wish to listen to our advice. Religion is advice.

## About The Author

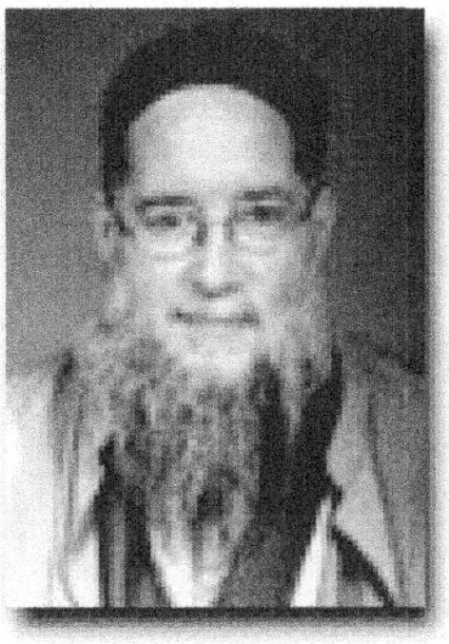

James McConnell

**James M. McConnell**, 'Sheikh Umar', was one of the first to offer information about hijama to the western and Internet audiences. From the start he has warned people about the influences that money would have on the ancient art of hijama. Now so many sites are attempting to turn hijama into a business. The healing arts are no more a business than religion is a business. A cleric is a weak servant of the people and does not enter the field of religion as a career choice or profession; he/she is called to serve. Selected, not elected.

Sheikh Umar McConnell, raised a Presbyterian, converted to Islam in 1992 and began his formal (book learning) Islamic education at the An-Nour Institute of Islamic Studies in Baltimore Maryland where he worked as an assistant Imam and participated in many interfaith programs. McConnell was the first student Imam to participate in the World Council of Churches, Seminaries Interacting Program. In

1999 McConnell was invited to attend the Imam and Khateeb program at Abu Nour University in Damascus Syria. He continued living and studying in Damascus with his wife and son for the next seven years.

McConnell continued his traditional, authorized education under the direct supervision of Sheikh Adnan Kabbani.

Sheikh Adnan often said;

*"Going to an Islamic University is beneficial only if at the end of your experience you realize that you have learned nothing at all"*

*He also often said;*

*"A real Islamic education does not come from books."*

He reminded his students that the Ilm (knowledge) of Prophet Muhammad (saw) was poured into the heart of Abu Bakr Siddiq, not memorized or learned.

McConnell received his ijaaza to practice Hijama in 2003 and has been credited as being one of the first to introduce hijama to the western world. He received his initial training working alongside **Sheikh Abu Bashar** in Damascus Syria, who has been providing hijama services free of charge to thousands of people over the past couple of decades. May Allah bless him for keeping this valuable sunnah of Prophet Muhammad (saws) alive and well.

*There is No Power and No Strength*

*Accept with the Creator*

بِسْمِ ٱللَّهِ ٱلرَّحْمَٰنِ ٱلرَّحِيمِ

In the Name of Allāh, the Most Gracious, the Most Merciful

# Table of Contents

## CHAPTER 1

**Glossary of Terms:**
**Ijaaza Isnad Matn Hadith Sunnah Harakat Qur'an Sunni Shi'a Sufism Mysticism Sheikh Dervish Iwan Halaqat Madrasa**

# Ijaaza System of Education

While most often attributed to the study of Quran and hadith, the ijaaza system of teaching in fact extends to all Islamic knowledge and disciplines. The history of the ijaaza system dates back before the time of the printing press. Hand written texts were carefully guarded in libraries, schools and places of worship. Memorization of texts was not sufficient alone to receive an Ijaaza as the text had to be committed to the heart as well as the mind. A hafiz of the Qur'an is a protector of the Qur'an and must have an intimate knowledge of the meaning and historical context to effectively protect the text. The ilm (knowledge) that Abu Bakr Siddiq received from Prophet Muhammad was poured into his heart, not his mind.

Who is one of the most proficient in memorizing the Qur'an backwards and forward? Shatan, the Devil.

A person must be pure to touch the Qur'an is thought to mean by most contemporary "scholars" that you must be ritualistically clean to pick up a Qur'an. While a minor meaning, the greater meaning is that you must be pure at heart to understand the deep spiritual and hidden meanings. A Qur'an in the hands of someone impure will in fact lead people further into disbelief. This is an important distinction that few understand today. In a similar manner, cupping practitioners who do not have a pure heart, no ijaaza, and practice for the sake of their own ego and Dunya (the material world) are leading themselves and others away from optimal spiritual and physical health.

Before a student was given the ijaaza for a specific text or subject material he or she had to demonstrate to a level of perfection not seen in education today the actual content (meaning) of the text as well as an understanding of the spirit and origin of the text or subject material.

With the dawn of Islam came an order from Allah (swt) to mankind to seek knowledge even if he had to go to China. In those days, "going to China to seek knowledge" meant seeking knowledge even to the "ends of the earth." Muslims took the order seriously and before the death of the Prophet (saw) they had the entire revelation of the Qur'an recorded in written form and there were many Muslims who had memorized the Qur'an entirely. They possessed the authorization to teach the oral recitation to others. Seeking knowledge even if you have to go to China was an order from Allah (swt) for all men and women to educate themselves in the prescribed manner of traditional learning. Up until that time only an elite few, mostly religious scholars, were educated in matters of reading, arithmetic, science and history. Muslims opened the way for education to spread from an elite few to the masses at large. Education of woman in the entire world was considered blasphemy and in some places punishable by death. Islam took away this oppression and several hundred years after common folk, male and female, were being educated in all matters in the Islamic world, women and commoners in Western Europe were still being persecuted by the Church for their desire to learn.

Even with the advent of expanded education for all, true scholars remained far and few between as the Ijaaza to convey or teach sacred knowledge was afforded only to those whose cleansing of the heart reached a point where their egos were under full control.

While Western Europe languished in the Dark Ages, the Middle East flourished under Islamic rule and this period is often referred to as the Golden Age of the Jews, which was in fact an age when the Jewish world was ruled by an Islamic Caliph and Sultan. The Muslims conquered Constantinople in the early 1300's (AD) and this cemented the power and rule of the Ottoman Empire over the Islamic region of the globe. By this time, the Madrasa had become the center for learning. These Islamic centers of learning dotted the Ottoman Empire which stretched from Persia over the entire Middle East through Turkey and into Eastern Europe. During that same time period in Western Europe the people languished in poverty to the point of eating their own dead. They lived in filth and were ravaged by the disease known as the Black Death, partly as a result of the poverty and filth in which they lived. The plague did touch the Middle and Far East, but it has long been recognized that because of the cleanliness of the Islamic lifestyle the toll on the Eastern world was not nearly as devastating as that of the West where over one-third of the population died. While the subjects, whether Muslim, Christian or Jew, living under Ottoman rule were given the freedom to live and educate themselves and deal in commerce unencumbered by governmental or religious oppression, the people of Western Europe struggled under the tyranny of the Catholic Church and the persecution of anyone who opposed it. When looking for an ideal societal model, one needs look no further than the Ottoman Empire, a vast region that at its peak of power was ruled by fewer than eighty government employees. People were educated in a manner whereby they governed themselves. Leaders were selected, not elected.

The revelation to "to read" came to an illiterate man named Muhammad (saws) who was orphaned as an infant, raised by a shepherd and his family, and who later went on to become a tradesman who led caravans of camels along the trade routes through the Arabian Desert. His goodness and qualification for prophet-hood and the receiving of the revelations later compiled and written down as the continuously existing Qur'an that we read today was inherent in his nature, not something he attained through education or something that was bestowed upon him by his clan for his excellence in business. He was selected by Allah (swt) from before the creation of the world to carry this revelation to the rest of us. Yet, he was sent to a lowly nation, was orphaned and shunned by his family as an outcast living with a sheep herding family on the outskirts of town. There was no more common a position in society as the one he held, and no lower station than that of an illiterate orphan. Before he was a prophet, Muhammad (saw) was a barefoot boy running with the sheep, playing with the other children, likely crying when he skinned his knee and comforted by the arms of the woman who was later called Hala Sultan, the Auntie of the Sultan. Just as Prophet Muhammad (saw) was selected to carry the greatest revelation ever to be bestowed on mankind, so too, students who carry on that knowledge are selected before leaving the Divine Presence on their journey to this earth. It is the responsibility of the authorized Teacher to determine whether this selection exists within the person he/she is teaching. When that inherent quality appears and the teacher knows the student has the moral fortitude and the strength of character required to carry the burden of the knowledge, then and only then does an ijaaza pass from the teacher to the student.

Just as not all students become teachers and not all citizens belong to the royal family, likewise not all those educated at the Madrasas of the Islamic Empire were given the title of Sheikh. Similarly, not all "Islamic scholars" who graduate from a modern day "Islamic University" are sheikhs or scholars and most are not connected through the true ijaaza system and cannot identify the isnad verifying their permission to pass on the knowledge they have gained or even identify the line of authorized sheikhs passing from their teachers back to Prophet Muhammad (saws). Many people claiming ijaaza today do not possess a qualified ijaaza with the proper isnad. It would be similar to creating a certificate from a major university you never actually attended or graduated from but rather obtained it from a student who failed to complete his studies or took one summer course at that same university – it's a fraud.

The sheikhs from the time of Prophet Muhammad (saw) up until this present day are those who were given the ijaaza by their sheikhs to carry the real banner of Islam from generation to generation. These sheikhs were and are, as Prophet Muhammad (saw) was, selected for their positions before they left Divine Presence and came to this earth. That selection was recognized by their Sheikh and once they were ready to carry their responsibility the banner was passed to them.

Between the Sunni, Shi'a and Sufi groups falling under the banner of Islam, the Sufi have traditionally maintained the Sunnah of oral transmission and the passing of an ijaaza from sheikh to student. The Sunni and Shi'a groups followed this system for many generations but have strayed far from the Sunnah in the last century. Sadly, most Sufi ways have also strayed from the real ijaaza system with students claiming false ijaaza on their sheikhs passing and those students bestowing ijaaza without real authorization. There is no such thing as shi'a, Sunni or Sufi designations in Islam and these titles only serve to divide believers from the true teachings of Prophet Muhammad (saws). Among the Jews, Christians and Muslims there are over two-hundred and twenty sects or denominations, among them only ONE is correct. It is the way of Imam Mehdi and Isa (Jesus), may the peace and blessings of Allah be upon them both. It is known in the Quran as the Rabbani Way. Ya Rab! Oh my Lord. For all of humanity who raise their hands and bow their heads in submission saying,"Oh my Lord." Welcome oh believers to the Rabbani Way!

The primary difference between a contemporary certificate or degree and an ijaaza is the tracing of the lineage of the knowledge or written text. Authorization to practice an art or transmit a written text or teach a body of knowledge within the ijaaza system is passed directly from a teacher to an individual student once that student demonstrates his or her competency and moral aptitude within the discipline or subject matter under study. There is no set program or timetable and no group graduations. Within the realm of Islamic studies this traceable lineage is called the isnad. The isnad is a traceable scholarly lineage back to the Prophet Muhammad (saws) going back through the companions through a subsequent line of authorized teachers.

For there to be an isnad, there must be a matn. The matn is the subject of the knowledge. Many people calling themselves Islamic scholars today cite the matn as a text (book), or even more broadly subject matter. They consider the texts of past scholars to be sources in and of themselves. The source for a true Islamic scholar is the Prophet (saw) himself. All other sources that cannot be traced back to the person of Prophet Muhammad (saws) are false innovations. These highly complicated texts and legalistic positions have brought about a generation of "Islamic Ulima" that have lost their connection with the Prophet (saw) and so have lost their legitimacy as leaders of the Muslim world. This unauthorized spiritually gutted approach to Islamic writings, including commentary found within translations of Qur'an and even the translations themselves, have resulted in a heavy burden which mankind is unable to carry and a face on the religion which looks more like the deformed face of the anti-Christ than the brilliant light of Prophet Muhammad's (saw) teachings. Schools of "Islamic Studies" today no longer carry the spiritual authority to pass on an ijaaza because they no longer carry the true flag of Rasool'allah, but have instead sold their golden reality for a bag of tin coins.

The true ijaaza system created a clear and succinct way to transmit information from one generation to the next. The contemporary study of written texts leaves too much to the individual for interpretation, then that one writes his or her interpretation and the old game of "Chinese whisper" goes quickly downhill with people pontificating opinions and claiming their writings are based on such and such or on the ancient writings of so and so. A strong ijaaza system has protected the written and recited Qur'an for the last 1433 years. Also protected by this system and then the tenacious efforts of those who prevent corruption of the old texts, has been the authenticated Hadith recordings of Sahi Muslim and Al Bukari. What, in our opinion, has lost legitimacy through the more modern and broken system, because the isnad has been all but lost, is the interpretation of these texts and the application of their meanings within society. Within the Islamic world the laws derived from the Qur'an and Hadith have been used to give lenience to the powerful and to constrict the meek. When a religion becomes a tool for oppression, we must conclude that the interpretation of that religious system has been taken over by unauthorized men who seek to gain power through the faith of the masses. Allah has clearly said that there is no compulsion in religion. If your religion keeps you from fulfilling your destiny then you are doing something wrong! Clearly, among the current Ulima calling themselves Sallafee and/or Wahabbi we find nothing of the spirit of Muhammad (saws) and much that resembles oppression.

An early scholar of Islam, Abdullah bin Mubarak, once said "Isnad is part of deen. If it were not for the sanad, then anyone would be able to say whatever they wished."

CHAPTER 2

**Glossary of Terms:**
**Doctorate University Conjecture**
**Baraka Ayat Dijal Shatan**
**Knowledge Justice**

# Western University and the Certification System

Without the isnad (lineage), knowledge quickly becomes mixed with opinion and conjecture, targeting products and services to a paying audience or customer base rather than protecting the divine information, trade, art and knowledge. Schools quickly succumb to market pressures, government propaganda, and effectively give students and the corrupt corporate industry what they want in exchange for the money they pay for a particular base of knowledge or degree. Colleges, universities and trade schools are nothing more than businesses selling diplomas. So many people want to know what they get for their money. What kind of certificate will I be guaranteed if I take your course, is one of the common demands people make. Effectively, asking the Sunnah of Rasool'allah to bow to the western university system.

Among the most ludicrous things I have read from Islamic historians and orientalists is this tendency to apologize for the rudimentary nature of the Islamic system of education. One example is a historian who will remain nameless, wrote that one of the great Madrasas of Egypt was recognized as being the closest to the modern day university because of its great lecture hall and the arrangement of its rooms - comparing the older to the newer, as if the older had been inspired by the newer system. Does that make sense? What that says is that the person making the comparison has no comprehension of true nobility and admires the spiritually dead modern system more than his own roots. So many Muslims today are ashamed of their own heritage, which is a rich and magnificent story! What is seen when looking at the old Madrasa compared to the new university is a weak attempt to capture the magnificence of the past. However hard they try they will never reach to the majesty of the past because they never had the connection. University halls today are lifeless money making institutions where students pay to be recognized. They turn students away from God and into debt slaves. The Islamic learning centers of the Golden age of Islam were centers of obedience to a command from Allah. They were centers for exploring and understanding the words of the Almighty Creator so that the student could better worship Allah and serve humanity. When the obedience and God consciousness leave an endeavor it loses its Baraka (divine blessing). There is no blessing in the modern university system, whether it is a university found in the east or the west. Those old Islamic schools that have traded reality for falsehood are doubly cursed because they have knowingly thrown the gifts given them by Allah (swt) behind their backs preferring profit rather than blessing, preferring Shatan to Allah (swt).

In like manner people are throwing Hijama behind their

backs for cupping, running after certification programs in a western environment and turning healing into cheating.

Young Muslims now pride themselves on their modern outlook and justify their seeking of degrees from these dead halls of regurgitation by quoting that Hadith which commands Muslims to seek knowledge even in China. They take this as justification for coming to a land which is clearly a land which has declared war on belief, whether Christian, Jew or Muslim, maintaining a moral lifestyle while living within the United States of America has become very difficult. Seeking acknowledgment for the regurgitation of empty useless knowledge is not the same thing as seeking knowledge. Most Muslim families are not satisfied if their sons and daughters choose to live simple lives learning a hand craft or farming. Most are not even satisfied with their children becoming teachers, or religious scholars. If shepherding was good enough work for the most beloved of Allah then why is it not good enough for your children? True knowledge brings wisdom. What these youth are learning today only brings chaos and confusion. The medical schools in today's universities are not educating health practitioners; they are indoctrinating soldiers for the dijal's army bringing ill health to all of mankind. Introducing illness through ineffective medicine to increase market share. Look at the board of directors at many of these cancer centers. A dear friend of mine who graduated from Harvard Law School many years ago said that he did not hear the word “justice” once as it applied to the actual application of the law, only as used in the context of revenge. If studying medicine does not train you to heal and studying law does not teach you to apply justice then what is the point of the studying? This is not the seeking knowledge that the Prophet spoke of. Rather it is a boosting of the ego with false knowledge and Shatanic pride, which we all know precedes a great fall.

The western certification or academic system while claiming to establish standards and practices that protect the integrity and excellence of a particular field or trade are more often than not nothing more than elaborate unions or associations that protect the financial interests of professionals who practice a given trade. The American Medical Association is one such example of a body that spends millions on lobbying efforts creating protectionist laws that benefit the professional and not the consumer or patient. In fact, this lobby has been so successful in protecting its trade in America that true healers are forbidden from practicing what is now labeled "alternative medicine." ObamaCare as written by insurance companies and will rapidly escalate prices while reducing available care. Euthanasia will become common. Prior to the 1920's doctors relied upon natural medicine until the Rockefeller's spent millions of dollars promoting pharmaceutical based medical practices.

Just as corporations have usurped the business world away from local businesses or sole proprietors, the corporate educational system has seized the age old apprentice educational model away from the accomplished and authorized master or teacher. This creates monopolistic educational enterprises that soon degrade the profession or trade and the industries to the point where they become focused primarily on profit rather than high moral standing and honor. Once accepted to a given certificate program the expectation is that if you achieve a certain academic score, regardless of your moral aptitude, you will receive a certificate for the money you paid. This system of producing tradesman, not students, has lost any sign of a moral compass and for this reason; people of integrity and faith should seek knowledge, as ordered by the Prophet (saws), even if they have to travel the world to find a true source.

CHAPTER 3

**Glossary of Terms:**
**Health Healer Homeopath Allopath Naturopath Osteopath Holistic Pharmaceutical Remedy Symptom Constitution**

# Natural Healing vs. Synthetic Treatment

When a child, still full of innocence and wonder at the world around them, decides that he or she wants to be a doctor it is usually because the child has an inherent desire to make sick people well. It comes from a nurturing nature and is often indicative of a calling to heal. The calling to be a healer used to be understood as just that, a calling, or an innate understanding of one's purpose on the planet. It was that persons act of worship. Recognizing this, they would seek out an authorized person to confirm their belief. Nowadays it seems to be based more on a need to dominate or control others, both intellectually and financially. The true healers of the past were the humble servants who traveled from house to house tending to those in their community whose bodies were ill or whose minds were out of synch. Today young men and women travel from every corner of the globe to attend prestigious medical schools in the west. Their families may spend the family fortune to put one child through these satanic medical schools. Do these families and individuals make this extraordinary effort and spend a family fortune on a calling to serve? In most cases, the answer is sadly, no. Having a "doctor" in the family is a status symbol. A medical degree is a prestigious degree. It is a position uplifting the ego, lordship, not true servanthood and certainly not that of a true healer. While there are always a few exceptions to the rule, nothing about medicine as it is practiced in the United States today is about true healing. The United States now ranks number 47th in the world for health care. Today, practicing medicine is just that, practicing with medication to cover symptoms that cause discomfort or disease. Just as covering a moldy wall with new boards and a fresh coat of paint does not cure the building of the toxic effects of the mold, so covering symptoms of illness within our bodies does not eliminate the dangerous disease of our system which can lead to the eventual destruction of the whole. Leaving some mold behind insures that there is plenty of business in the future.

The first medical association formed in the United States was the American Institute for Homeopathy formed in 1844 after the rise in popularity of homeopathy among the countries elite citizens. In 1846 the American Medical Association formed mainly in defense of what they perceived as an encroachment of homeopathy treatment on their territory. The American Medical Association admitted only "traditional" or medication based doctors to its membership and strictly forbid membership to homeopaths. By the beginning of the twentieth century the life's blood had been squeezed out of the homeopathy movement in America and the American Medical Association had all but won. Today, in order to practice homeopathy in the United States one must first submit themselves to the indoctrination of what we have coined the medical mafia, or the standards and practices of the American Medical Association, by completing four years of pre-med and at least four years of medical school.

Medical School in the United States, Britain and most of the United Kingdom is more an indoctrination into a very narrow symptom based set of rules rather than a real education in the physiology and care of the human being. It has become solely a study of the body systems as though each of us were made from the same mold. The only answers are expensive drugs to treat this symptom, then another expensive drug to treat the symptom caused by the first drug. For the most part drugs in the allopathic pharmacopeia are synthetically altered chemicals designed to block certain functions in order to control symptoms. This design as a path to healing seems ludicrous from a scientific point of view, because blocking a natural action within the body to alleviate one symptom is bound to do damage to another system causing more problems which require more drugs to control those symptoms. If a car mechanic corrected a problem in your car by using a fluid or application that damaged another part of your car requiring that you come back again for further repair and then did this over and over again, you would accuse him of unfair business practices. When challenged that there is a natural fluid that is free for the taking and causes no damage at all, the mechanic would tell you that fluid is not recommended or certified. How much more heinous is this when it is our very lives, rather than just our car, that is being destroyed?

An allopathic doctor once said to me that allopathic literally means "against nature." He was responding to my many concerns about the prescriptions he offered as the only solutions to my illness. He stated, "this is what we allopathic doctors do! We prescribe drugs." When I asked him about the side effects he said that he would find something for me to take to counteract the side effects. This idea seemed preposterous to me. Certainly there was a way to lower my cholesterol without risking the possibility of permanent muscle and liver damage! Some may say that a more accurate translation of the term allopathic is "against suffering." Whatever the actual translation, it has come to represent doctors who treat symptoms with pharmaceutical drugs. They read numbers on lab or blood test and gauge their prescription of synthetic chemicals based on those numbers and charts which they have been taught represent the state of human health. The actual term "allopathic" was coined by C.F.S. Hahnemann to designate the usual practice of medicine as opposed to homeopathy.

Homeopathy is an intricate system of energy based remedies which create within the body a positive resonant energy resulting in restoration. This is simply the opposite of the negative energy response created within an atom that results in explosion or destruction. When the molecular structure of the atom is split, or destroyed, that destruction carries on producing the explosion that all of mankind has come to fear. So, to say that energy cannot expand having an effect on the molecules around it is simply ignorance and a denial of science. Nobody questions that the atomic bomb is a negative energy based reaction that causes horrendous destruction. Why then do many scientists ignore and many people question the possibility that positive energy resonance can expand in a positive and restorative manner within the human body?

Homeopathy, using the properties of energy resonance, operates under the premise that a symptom is evidence of a deficiency or need within the body for balance. The idea that using the very property that seems to have caused the disease, broken down into minute energy molecules, will then expand upon themselves and fill the deficiency thus relieving the body of the symptom. Unlike pharmaceuticals which cover the symptom from the outside, homeopathic remedies begin at the molecular level to heal from the inside out. The symptom is relieved because it is no longer needed to warn the body of the deficiency within itself. There is no danger from the use of homeopathic remedies because the substance from which the energy has been derived has been reduced to its minute energy level and can no longer be distinguishable as a component of the remedy. Meaning there is no identifiable substance found within the remedy liquid or tablet. The tablets are sugar tablets and the water is simply water. The remedy itself is at the molecular level containing only the energy of the original substance. Further, the original substances used are naturally based and thus are easily incorporated into the natural foundation for the remedy, be it tablet or liquid and are thus energetically compatible with the human body. Chemically based pharmaceuticals are synthetics which do not ever completely conform to the energy base of our human body and thus are poison, even in minute amounts.

Homeopathy treats the entire person as one being. An initial consultation with a true homeopath can take a few hours as the doctor gathers information from every aspect of the patient's life experiences and responses. It is not prone to becoming rich. Once the doctor is familiar with the patient then remedies can be prescribed more readily when problems and illness arise. A person may need to take a constitutional remedy to bring their being back into balance before more difficult problems can be addressed. Homeopathic healing is a process. Your body did not get into a bad energy state in one instance or with one bad experience and it will not balance itself again with only one application or treatment. In homeopathy patience is important as restoration begins deep and moves outward slowly.

In summary, homeopathy has its foundation and works off the principles of the energy of life having the power to heal when stimulated in a positive manner to do so. An allopathic method simply studies the visible destruction and does its best to cover the ugliness of the destruction but does nothing to cure the destroying property underneath.

It is clear which of the two makes logical sense. When it comes to reattachment of a severed limb or necessary surgical procedures, allopathic medicine excels and has its place in the overall medical industry. Its dominance and control over the medical field, however, has become destructive to overall health.

As more people become aware of the destructive properties of synthetic pharmaceuticals they are waking up to the reality that what they once perceived as the best medical system in the world is really just a profit driven industry and that their lives are the fuel which feeds it. That industry has, from its inception in the mid 1880's, been driven by greed and the desire to dominate the profit shares of a never ending market. Everyone dies and everyone fears, or at least resists, death. Promises to cure people have always brought a following. Now, in the twenty-first century that market share has been dominated and controlled by the AMA, a group that we equate to modern mafia groups that hold a population hostage forcing unprotected people to tolerate their oppression and control for the sake of monetary profit. They know their methods create more disease, but it fits their business model and increases overall profits.

Homeopaths have been dismissed by this group as quacks and many doctors who are truly called to be healers have fought the many entanglements of the AMA only to be subjugated to censor and threatened with expulsion from the practice of medicine altogether. In a desperate effort to bring about a more holistic approach to the practice of medicine, these doctors have formed groups which have gained some recognition within the medical community controlled by the AMA mafia. These two groups of doctors are called osteopaths and naturopaths. These groups approach the study of medicine from the perspective of the patient as a whole person rather than as separate parts or systems. The naturopath incorporates more natural approaches to healing which can include what is now termed alternative medicine. However, both are required to complete a graduate program in medicine which is approved by the AMA and both are required to perform a residency in a medical hospital environment. In order to practice homeopathy in the United States one must have a title from one of these disciplines first. Meaning the student must sell themselves to the idea that energy resonant healing is quackery before they are then permitted to practice it!

CHAPTER 4

**Glossary of Terms:**
**Hadith Cure Chronic Illness**
**Genetically modified food**
**Environmental contamination**
**Cellular oxygenation**

# Hijama, A Cure for All Illness

As Muslims, our superior method of Prophetic sayings protected by a unique science of hadith system and the Ijaaza process that requires an isnad back to Prophet Muhammad (saws) is the best assurance and protection we have that hijama is a favored and effective treatment for all illness. All healing comes from Allah (swt), correct belief therefore, is the basis of all healing. Conforming to the purpose for which you were created results in perfect health. One should work eight hours per day, sleep eight hours per day and pray eight hours per day. The Sahaba (first followers) of Prophet Muhammad (saw) rarely went to a doctor as illnesses were almost completely eradicated.

**Most illness comes to shock you back into the reality of your REAL existence, or to bring you to your grave.**

To join in the western profit motivated and often corrupt system of clinical trials and studies to prove Hijama as an effective treatment is in large part denying the Prophetic tradition and stepping away from our Islamic practice. The current medical model has clearly failed to eradicate illness and disease. The rates of chronic illnesses are off the charts with a thousand fold increases or more in cases of cancer, high blood pressure, diabetes, kidney failure, and the list goes on and on. Following the current "scientific" western model should consequently be seen as an absurd path or model to pursue, not an example to emulate.

During the time of Prophet Muhammad (saws) there were very few illnesses that man suffered from. When becoming sick a person would either get well within a few days or die a rather quick death. There were very few, if any, long term chronic conditions that people suffered from. Illnesses have increased as our disobedience and disbelief has become more stubborn. For a person to come in and ask if Hijama will cure such and such is in effect disbelief. Asking, does Hijama cure this condition or that condition, is to begin the healing process by first denying what the Prophet (saws) said about Hijama being a cure for all illness and God being at the root of all cures. No, Hijama will not cure you, but properly attributed to Allah, it will cure everything. How we see illness in the west is upside down.

With that said . . . . A Cure for All Illness? How is Hijama a Cure for All Illness?

First and foremost, we must clarify that we are primarily speaking about naturally occurring illness and disease when we say cupping is a cure for all illness. If your arm is severed, Hijama will not cause you to grow another arm, but it will aid in the healing process when reattaching a limb. So we must first separate conditions resulting from unnatural causes from actual illnesses. Kidneys destroyed by environmental contamination, pharmaceutical side effects, or genetically modified foods, will not be restored with Hijama. Compromised kidneys however would benefit greatly from hijama therapy, helping to stop or slow down the disease process by, in large part, providing optimal delivery of oxygen, nutrients and hydration to your organs so they can fight the disease and illness affecting them. People must therefore seek to eliminate the cause of the root illness as well. A trained and authorized Hijama practitioner should be knowledgeable about the many factors that are destroying people's good health and help clients to follow a plan to reduce or eliminate these factors. They should also be able to identify weaknesses in worship and how to instruct people to get right with God. Thikr (meditation) is critically important in achieving optimal health.

The body God gave us is cured by permission from God alone. God has nonetheless provided our body an amazing ability to cure itself. Hijama effectively enhances the body's ability to cure itself by optimizing the pathways that deliver the essential elements we need to be healthy and strong. Modern medical practices rarely address the cause of illness and often only provide a synthetic or artificial cure, which is not a real cure at all. It normally results in adverse health effects and more stubborn illness. Surgery, often unnecessary, takes years off your life and most often could have been avoided with good preventative measures such as Hijama.

Oxygen, food and water are the essentials of all physical life.

One can survive weeks without food, and several days without water, but remove oxygen for more than a few minutes and life ends. The cardiovascular system is responsible for distributing the air, food and water we consume to the entire body. Thousands of miles of arteries, veins and capillaries keep our bodies alive and well, distributing vital oxygen, nutrients and hydration to all the life giving cells. We know what happens if we stop all oxygen to our body... we die; but what happens when oxygen to our organs is hampered by years of neglect, sedentary lives, poor diet, artificial food, and the enormous amounts of environmental contaminants we are exposed to each and every day of our lives? The answer is easily understood; our bodies die slowly.

Hijama removes dead blood cells in the cardiovascular system that otherwise would impede the body's ability to heal itself. In this manner it is in fact a cure for all natural illness caused by the reduction of oxygen, nutrients and hydration reaching vital organs and cells. Therefore, to properly clean the cardiovascular system you must educate yourself and understand how to avoid the many toxins in our environment. Then practice the tradition of Hijama as prescribed by the Sunnah to cleanse dead refuse from your blood and change the water inside your body with positive energy resonance by performing thikr Allah, and you will likely enjoy a very long and disease free life.

**The root of all good health is belief in the Creator of All Things, full stop.**

Hijama is by far the most important thing you can perform

to maintain good health - evidence by the explosion of interest in Hijama therapy. Ten years ago it was virtually unknown in the West. Hijama has become even more important as the list of things harming us grows each day. We all understand the importance of good diet and exercise, but if our bodies are effectively clogged up from years of neglect and environmental toxins, exercise and diet alone will not help. You can put anti-freeze and clean water in your radiator, but if it does not circulate well, the car will overheat. The same holds true with our body.

Our assertion is that Hijama is a far better method to oxygenate the body than current oxygen therapy methods. Therefore, a review of the benefits of oxygen therapy might be informative in determining the overall benefits of Hijama treatment. Different varieties of oxygen therapy are promoted as alternative treatments for dozens of diseases, including certain types of cancer, asthma, emphysema, AIDS, arthritis, heart and vascular diseases, multiple sclerosis, and Alzheimer's disease. Oxygen therapy is said to have a positive effect on the overall health because it increases the efficiency of all cells in the body and increases (really changes) energy, promotes the production of antioxidants, and enhances the immune system.

There is significant evidence that cancer cells thrive in low-oxygen environments. It is said that adding oxygen to the body creates an oxygen-rich condition in which cancer cells cannot survive. In order to understand the dramatic effect of increased oxygenation on cancer it is important to explain the conditions which allow cancer cells to not only survive but multiply and flourish. We are speaking about the oxygenation on a cellular level so we are going to look at the metabolism which occurs on a cellular level.

A normal healthy cell functions aerobically, which means it needs oxygen to metabolize. A well functioning aerobic cell burns oxygen and glucose for energy and releases carbon dioxide in an efficient manner. Anaerobic cells, cells which flourish in a low oxygen or absent oxygen environment cannot thrive there. This includes cancer, Epstein Barr, herpes, mono, genital warts, and most viruses.

An unhealthy or diseased cell is lacking sufficient oxygen but will still produce energy by burning mainly protein. This is very inefficient and a severe strain on the bodies organs and muscles. This energy burning process releases mainly lactic acid and carbon monoxide instead of carbon dioxide. This cell is functioning anaerobically - with no oxygen present. Cancer and viral diseases flourish in this environment.

Therefore, anaerobic cells burn much more glucose to produce the same amount of energy as aerobic. Cancer cells exhibit this anaerobic mode of metabolism - lack of oxygen, high glucose consumption, carbon monoxide and high lactic acid production. Cancer cells thrive in this high sugar-low oxygen environment but cannot exist in the opposite condition of high oxygen-low sugar mode of healthy cells.

In "The Prime Cause and Prevention of Cancer" published in 1967 by a Dr. Otto Warburg, these facts about cancer and the oxygenation of cells was explored and found to have great significance in the treatment and cure of cancer in the human body. His findings have been unjustifiably minimized by the medical mafia. Dr Warburg was a biochemist in cancer research. He won the Nobel Prize in Medicine for proving that cancer cannot exist in an oxidizing, healthy cell. Dr. Warburg was the director of the Max Planck Institute for Cell Physiology in Germany.

Dr. Warburg proposed that normalizing the metabolism of cancer cells was the key to effective cancer treatment and the means to accomplish this was to increase the oxygen content of the cells. Dr. Warburg stated that as the first priority of treatment, "-- all growing body cells be saturated with oxygen" and the second priority was to avoid further exposure to toxins. Such a simple solution and now so many years later the medical mafia and their pharmaceutical partners are still creating new toxic poisons to kill cancer cells and good cells alike. Just another proof that if it doesn't make money the medical mafia is not interested in the cure.

There has been successful treatment and cure of herpes zoster in many European countries using the injection of ozone/oxygen. When the doctor says cure, he is following the standard for cancer in that five years disease free qualifies as a cure. In a study performed by a Dr. R. Mattassi at the Santa Corona Hospital in Milan, Italy 90% of patients treated with intravenous injections, from one to five injections only, were still relapse free five years later. It was suspected that the remaining 10% were reinfected, not relapsed. Cuba, Russia, and West Germany have also successfully treated viral infections, such as herpes zoster, with increased oxygenation. At the Center of Medical and Surgical Research in Havana, fifteen adult patients suffering from herpes zoster were treated with injections of ozone/oxygen for a period of fifteen days. All patients were completely symptom free after the treatment and follow-up examinations a year later showed not one relapse.

Sufficient amounts of increased oxygenation at the cellular level kill the herpes virus. Further, Herpes virus infection is at epidemic levels in the United States. However, ozone/oxygen therapy is not an FDA approved treatment for herpes. If they are doing experiments with it, it certainly is not available to the masses. Could that be because simple oxygen therapy is not patentable? Therefore, no company is willing to spend five to seven years and millions of dollars obtaining FDA approval when they cannot recoup their expenditures. Just more evidence that our medical system is not based on what is good for the people but what is good for business. The good news is that we don't need a patent or millions of dollars worth of research to tell you that Hijama can and does help deliver oxygen to the body at a cellular level by flushing the system of dead blood cells and rejuvenating the cardiovascular system. As the popularity of Hijama grows it will come under increasing attacks by the AMA and the FDA. It is, however, a religious procedure protected by the constitution; which we all now see being dismantled before our eyes.

Our environment is becoming more and more toxic as our governments spray aluminum and barium dust over our heads and allow corporations to fill our food with synthetic materials and sell them as nutritious. We all suffer from a lack of oxygen - even those who exercise daily. If you live in America in 2013 then you are suffering from a lack of oxygen and this lack of oxygen is slowly killing us all. The weak and already sick among us will die off first but don't be fooled into thinking that because you eat fruits and vegetables and watch your weight and run every day that you are not going to succumb to the poisons that we are exposed to everyday. Your cells are being deprived of oxygen, a component for life. Hijama twice a year as a precaution can help curb the effects of this bombardment, but we all have to make some changes in the way we live if we hope to live to become old.

**Here is what some experts have to say on oxygenation.**

**On Breathing and Good Health**

"Improper breathing is a common cause of ill health. If I had to limit my advice on healthier living to just one tip, it would be simply to learn how to breathe correctly. There's no single more powerful - or simpler - daily practice to further your health and well-being than breathwork." ~ Andrew Weil, M.D. In his book, Breathing: The Master Key to Self-Healing.

"Breathing is the key that unlocks the whole catalog of advanced biological function and development. Is it any wonder that it is so central to every aspect of health? Breathing is the first place, not the last, one should look when fatigue, disease, or other evidence of disordered energy presents itself. Breathing is truly the body's most basic communication system." Sheldon Saul Hendler, MD, Ph.D. Oxygen Breakthrough, p. 96

I remind myself and the reader that meditation (thikr Allah) is vital for good health, not only from the point of energy resonance but from the breathing techniques it induces.

**On Cancer**

"The first discovery was made by Nobel Prize winner Dr. Otto Warburg, Director of the Max Planck Institute for Cell Physiology in Berlin. He confirmed that the key precondition for the development of cancer is a lack of oxygen at the cellular level." ~Nathaniel Altman(Oxygen Healing Therapies, Pg. 66.)

"Lack of oxygen clearly plays a major role in causing cells to become cancerous." ~Dr. Harry Goldblatt,(Journal of Experimental Medicine )

"Cancer has only one prime cause. It is the replacement of normal oxygen respiration of the body's cells by an anaerobic (ie., oxygen-deficient) cell respiration."~Dr. Otto Warburg

"Cancer is a condition within the body where the oxidation has become so depleted that the body cells have degenerated beyond physiological control. Similarly, the true cause of allergy is lowered [sic] the oxidation process within the body, causing the affected individual to be sensitive to foreign substances entering the body. Only when the oxidation mechanism is restored to its original high state of efficiency can the sensitivity be eliminated." ~ Dr. Wendell Hendricks, (Two-time Nobel Laureate, Winner of the Nobel Prize for Cancer Research, Hendricks Research Foundation)

**On Detoxification**

"Many healings of other physical troubles have occurred in my clients after they started to integrate breathing practices into their lives. There is a simple but encompassing reason that may explain this. The human body is designed to discharge 70% of its toxins through breathing. Only a small percentage of toxins are discharged through sweat, defecation and urination. If your breathing is not operating at peak efficiency, you are not ridding yourself of toxins properly." ~Gay Hendricks, PhD Conscious Breathing, Pg. 17.

## On Anxiety, Panic

Fear is excitement without the breath. ~Fritz Perl, M.D. Founder of Gestalt Therapy.

On Asthma

"One study on the treatment of asthma patients conducted by researchers John Goyeche, Dr. Ago, and Dr. Ikemi, suggests that any effective treatment should address suppressed emotions - such as anxiety and self-image - as well as the physical dimension. To achieve this, they encourage correction of poor posture, and helping the person relax the irrelevant respiratory muscles while restoring full diaphragmatic breathing. They also recommended finding ways for getting rid of excess mucus. The good news is that a well-rounded breath practice will do all these things." ~ Donna Farhi (The Breathing Book, Pg. 207)

## On Blood Pressure

"The relationship between breathing and blood pressure has been known and understood for a long time. It boils down to this: Elevated blood pressure accompanies those bodily states where rapid shallow breathing prevails. By altering breathing to a slow diaphragmatic mode, blood pressure decreases."~ Robert Fried, PhD (The Breath Connection, Pg. 152.)

**On Heart Disease**

"Coronary heart disease is due to a lack of oxygen received by the heart." ~Dr. Dean Ornish

"...healthy breathing should be the first thing taught to a heart patient. A Dutch Study conducted by a Dr. Dixhoorn, compared two groups of heart attack patients. The first group was taught simple diaphragmatic breathing, while the second group was given no training in breathing. The breathing group had no further heart attacks, while 7 of the 12 members of the second group had second heart attacks over the next 2 years."~ Gay Hendricks, Ph.D. (Conscious Breathing, Pg. 16).

"A lack of oxygen (hypoxia) is the prime cause of 1.5 million heart attacks each year."~ Dr. Richard Lippman, Renowned researcher

**On the Lymphatic System**

"Jack Shield, MD, a Lymphologist from Santa Barbara, CA, conducted a study on the effects of breathing on the lymphatic system. Using cameras inside the body, he found that deep diaphragmatic breathing stimulated the cleansing of the lymph system by creating a vacuum effect which sucked the lymph through the bloodstream. This increased the rate of toxic elimination by as much as 15 times the normal pace."~ "Lymph, Lymph Glands, and Homeostasis"25 No. 4, Dec 92, Pg.147-153

**On Overcoming Disease**

"All chronic pain, suffering, and diseases are caused by a lack of oxygen at the cell level." Dr. Arthur C. Guyton, M.D, author The Textbook on Medical Physiology.

"Breathing is the key that unlocks the whole catalog of advanced biological function and development. Is it any wonder that it is so central to every aspect of health? Breathing is the first place, not the last, one should look when fatigue, disease, or other evidence of disordered energy presents itself. Breathing is truly the body's most basic communication system." ~ Sheldon Saul Hendler, MD, PhD. (Oxygen Breakthrough, Pg 96)

"Oxidation is the source of life. Its lack causes impaired health or disease, its cessation, death." ~ Dr. F.M. Eugene Blass, PH.D., (Oxygen Therapy: Its Foundation, Aim, Results)

"Oxygen plays a pivotal role in the functioning of the immune system."Parris M. Kidd, Ph.D. author, Antioxidant Adaption

"Starved of oxygen, the body will become ill, and if this persists it will die, I doubt if there is an argument about that." ~ Dr. John Muntz, Nutritional Scientist

"Insufficient oxygen means insufficient biological energy that can result in anything from mild fatigue to life-threatening disease. The link between insufficient oxygen and disease has now been firmly established."~ W. Spencer Way, (Journal of the American Association of Physicians)

"Cells undergoing partial oxygen starvation send out tiny panic signals which are collectively felt in the body as a continuous vague sensation of uneasiness, dread or disaster. This low level generalized warning tends to get tuned out as mere "background noise" by the individual experiencing it. Or, it is attributed to other sources of uneasiness... People rarely suspect that the constant vague feelings of helplessness, fatigue... uneasiness are symptoms of cellular oxygen deprivation."Excerpted from Townsend Letter for Doctors.

CHAPTER 5

## Glossary of Terms:
## Eugenics Cure Chronic Illness
## Genetically modified food
## Environmental contamination

# Sick By Design

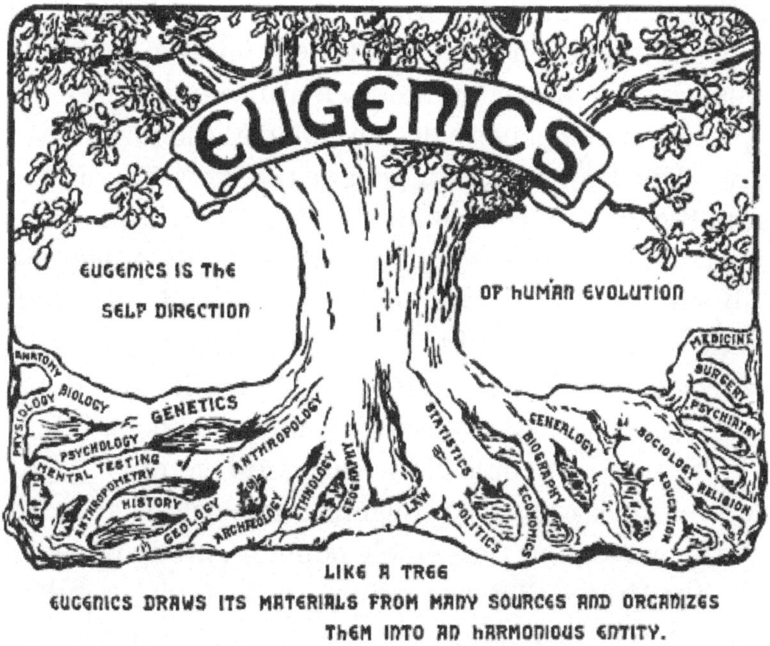


Logo of the Second International Congress of Eugenics.

The Second International Exhibition of Eugenics held September 22 to October 22, 1921, in connection with The Second International Congress of Eugenics in the American

Museum of Natural History, New York (Baltimore: William & Wilkins Co., 1923).

Eugenics was taught and studied in the late nineteenth century and early to mid-twentieth century. It became the foundation for Hitler's ideologies and the catalyst for the Second World War. Eugenics teaches that the "evolution" of mankind as a species can be self directed, or manipulated. What does that mean? Eugenics is the scientifically researched and pursued efforts to eliminate those that the founders, directors and their descendants deem to be inferior. If you and your ancestors were not included in their superior group, then you are slated for elimination. This is an established area of documented scientific study based on an interpretation of a genetic theory called Mendelian Inheritance. The framework for genetic theory was first taken from the work of Gregor Johann Mendel whose work was published in 1865 and 1866. Around 1900 the Eugenics idea of directed evolution was born from this understanding that genetic inheritance could be manipulated to create a human species of the smartest, the most beautiful and the strongest. These views were supported and propagated by some very influential people of the early 20th century. The first International Congress of Eugenics was held in 1912. At that time the movement was widely popular among the elite families in the United States and Europe. However, as full comprehension of the magnitude of these ideas became clear in the minds of the God fearing these ideas became very controversial and supposedly the Eugenics programs were all but discontinued in the mid 1940's. However it is clear that those who had visions of a pure human species did not cease to pursue their goals.

Despite the concerted efforts to make the world believe that the Eugenics movement is a thing of the past, Eugenics is very much alive and well in the world today, virtually dominating the western scientific and educational institutions. While high school history books attribute the eugenics movement primarily to Nazi Germany and their favored eugenic method of extermination of the inferior species of humans, the eugenics movement actually was conceived of in the American scientific community and is still very prevalent in scientific circles today. It is an extremely sophisticate scientifically based attack on the population to cull the masses – rid the world of useless eaters. It is now done secretly by adding components to your diet, water, air that target certain populations, mainly the poor who are forced to buy their food from big box discount stores.

In the deep and varied writings on the subject one finds three main categories or methods of applying Eugenics to a human population. The first is a eugenics program mandated on a population, much like the oppressive restrictions and controls placed on the populations in China and North Korea over the last decades. The second is presented as promotional voluntary eugenics. This sounds like a positive but really with the control of our media from the inception of radio and television, it is not really voluntary because there is no informed consent. Promotional voluntary eugenics is just another way accomplishing their goal while allowing the masses to think that they have made good decisions for themselves. This was the course of the eugenics movement throughout the remainder of the 20th century. They did not give up their aspirations for a pure human species; they simply took a route that allowed the masses to believe they were safe. The last form discussed is called private eugenics in which the philosophies are practiced voluntarily within a group of individuals but not promoted to the general population. This third form is reserved for the elite globalists and their offspring as they have worked over the decades to create their super species.

Now, in the early 21st century, these globalist eugenicists have infiltrated every level of our world government. Something not well understood is the depths of the second form of eugenics where populations have been manipulated through extensive promotional bombardment by eugenics/governments/corporations to believe that certain poisonous agents in their food, air, water and medicine supply are actually for their benefit. This is where we wish to emphasis the "Sick by Design" intentional attacks perpetrated upon humanity for the purpose of reducing undesirable populations. The eugenics movement no longer distinguishes between races as much as they do genetically inferior populations which transcend race and religious groups. While race is still a factor it has become more a general emphasis on reducing the total number of "useless eaters" within the population. Who are the "useless eaters", you and I, for the most part? The modern eugenics movements stated goals, from leading members like Henry Kissinger, Bill Gates and Ted Turner in many white papers written over the past two decades is to reduce world populations by more than eighty percent.

Why is this relevant and necessary in a book about Hijama? The vast majority of the patients coming to alternative practitioners are people who are under full blown attack from this modern eugenics movement. The populations are being culled. The general belief or public relations message the eugenics movement wishes to convey is that overpopulation is the biggest threat to mankind and that responsible (superior) people need to manage, really control, the populations. Greed and power is the driving force behind this movement, not a concern for humanity, as everyone already knows, if populations did exceed numbers that the earth could support, natural forces (God) would reduce world populations naturally. Who gives anyone the right to determine who lives and who dies, the eugenics movement today feels they are best equipped to determine the fate of the world's populations. Making themselves out to be on the level of God, while in fact serving their master Satan (Shatan). With this belief they have systematically begun to cull the world's populations through many different scientific and regulatory methods. They believe they derive power from killing people and feed from the anger or negative energy it creates. This is just one reason why Thikr (meditation) is critical in achieving whole health as it provides positive energy force to combat the negative energy force - light vs. darkness.

Evidence that this movement was thriving and working undercover throughout the 20th century became public again in 1993 with the unveiling of UN Agenda 21 program. They openly began this worldwide effort to reduce populations and return the world to a pre-industrialized state. At the core is a plan to establish a "new world order," one world governing body that would regulate all human activity primarily through carbon emissions and other global regulatory schemes that are being once again promoted as being for our own safety and protection.

Now that their "super species" is intact, and robotics can replace the armies and work forces, it is time to increase the volume of the poisons in the food, air and water on the populations to be eliminated. Over the last two decades, since the turn of the century, rates of chronic illness have skyrocketed. Autism in children has increased from 1 in 25,000 twenty years ago to 1 in 80 and plummeting! Vaccines mandated for America's children have gone from three to four injections twenty years ago to over thirty injections by the time children reach kindergarten! Can we see a correlation there? Have there been studies to research this correlation? Pharmaceutical companies are developing more and more synthetic drugs and marketing them to the population with extensive warnings, yet the population is so brain dead from so many contaminates that they run to their doctors asking for more poison! Obesity is off the charts with young people in their twenties suffering from weight related terminal illness. Can you say Dijal 101 (the anti-Christ)?

**Here are just a few of their soft kill weapons of choice.**

**Sodium fluoride** widely dispersed in the US water system causes sterility and cancer as well as reducing IQ's. In 2006, a study published in The Lancet identified fluoride as "an emerging neurotoxin substance" that causes severe brain damage. The National Research Council (NRC) wrote that "it is apparent that fluorides have the ability to interfere with the functions of the brain and the body by direct and indirect means."

Two of the pioneers in bringing attention to the public about the dangers of fluoride in water are infowars.com and NaturalNews.com. A rather exhaustive body of work on the subject can be found by searching these websites.

**Biosphenol A** in the plastic food and drink containers causes increased rates of cancer and sterility, Biosphenol A, also called BPA was used in the 1930's to enhance the growth of cattle and poultry. It is likely still used for this purpose in many parts of the world. It is a dangerous practice which puts the public at severe risk of cancer and sterility. It was also used as an estrogen replacement for women. Recognizing the dangers of its use in women it was quickly discontinued as an estrogen replacement. Based on research by chemists at Bayer and General Electric, BPA has been used since the 1950s to harden polycarbonate plastics and make epoxy resin, and in the lining of food and beverage containers. So, the substance was not approved for use as an estrogen replacement as early as the 1930's yet it has been used for years in the plastics industry without regulation. It wasn't until 1997 when evidence of a correlation began to emerge between exposure to BPA and estrogen related diseases like breast cancer and sterility. It has been replaced by BPS, which is now found to be worse than BPA.

Currently there are no BPA or BPS labeling requirements for plastics.

**High Fructose Corn Syrup** increases your risk of obesity, diabetes, hypertension, liver damage and mercury poisoning. According to current research this may have much more to do with the GMO nature of most of the corn rather than from the corn itself. Meaning, if we could derive the sugar from organic non GMO corn we may not see the devastating effects seen from "modern" corn syrup.

**GMO Food Products-** We could go deep into the science and studies showing GMO food products to be dangerous for human consumption, but it is sufficient to make it known that the scientists working at Monsanto have placed in their own contracts that genetically modified foods cannot be served inside their own company's cafeteria. If the scientists who created GMO food products will not consume GMO food products, neither should anyone else. Search the internet for "Dangers of GMO Food Products."

**Vaccines-**The original science of vaccination made sense. The scientific foundation actually sounds very similar to the like cures like principles of homeopathy. A little of a bad virus developed an immunity against that same virus when it came around with a vengeance. This seemed like a huge scientific step forward for populations devastated by polio and measles in the mid 20th century. However, as people of evil intention often do, eugenicists have taken this valuable scientifically based technology and have used it for their own evil agenda. There is no shortage of research regarding the negative effects of a wide variety of vaccines on the market today. The entire industry has been usurped. There are no safe vaccines anymore. From Gardisil to the seasonal flu shot, studies have proven that the extreme risks associated with vaccinating oftentimes outweigh the minor benefits. For a more exhaustive review of articles and studies related to the dangers of vaccines see our reference page at the end of this book.

**"Chemtrails"- Chemical trails seen in the skies over our heads.** Statistical evidence shows that lung issues such as asthma and COPD have risen considerably over the past two decades. Trails of aluminum barium sulphate are falling on the heads of you, your children, your farm animals and your gardens. For more information watch the 2012 critically acclaimed documentary, "Why in the World are They Spraying" and draw your own conclusions.

Hijama practitioners must stay current with these and other trends in an effort to help educate patients about the many environmental factors harming people. This book is not intended to be an exhaustive authority on the subject, only to call attention to factors that often need to be addressed with patients seeking health assistance and spiritual guidance. Educating patients about proper nutrition and teaching methods on how to avoid the many poisonous agents encountered in their daily lives is critical in providing people with overall health advice. Hijama treatment will certainly help restore the health of those suffering from these environmental attacks, but unless the practitioner addresses the underlining causes the patient will continue to suffer.

Infowars.com, prisonplanet.com, rense.com, healthranger.com and naturalnews.com are just a few good resources that may help keep the reader up to date about what is happening to combat these assaults on the human population.

CHAPTER 6

## Glossary of Terms:
## Energy resonance Thikr Meditation Spirituality Awlia

# Importance of Spirit, Water and Meditation

Mankind was made from the clay of the earth. What is clay? A fraction of parts water and a fraction of parts earth, correct? If man was fashioned from clay and simply given the breath of life would his body not be more densely earth than water? Why then do you suppose that man's body is on average 70% water? Why is the fraction of earth so greatly reduced from that of hard sticky clay, from which he was first molded? What gives the human being his buoyancy? From where does the water of life flow?

From within water, flows the property of life itself. Without water, there is no life, full stop. On this planet all living things require water and are made of a percentage of water. So it goes to reason that the force we call life is somehow embodied within this thing we call water. So, then begs the question. What is water? Well, chemically water is 2 molecules of hydrogen balanced with 1 molecule of oxygen. Just as the body requires the respiration of it for life, so the cell, on a molecular level, requires the existence of it for survival.

The element that literally gives life to all living things is Oxygen – the O in H2O. Oxygen is invisible, it has no taste, no smell; we cannot feel it or hear it. Yet we believe in it and without it we will die. Without it the entire existence of life on this planet will cease to be. So, is it then the property of "Being"?

What is the shape of water? Does it restrain itself to a location or to limits? What are the properties of water that make it something which can live within us, outside of us, in and on all earth surfaces and where does it go when it evaporates? Does it cease to exist? Ever? Or does it regroup and come back down on us as rain; life giving rain. Its bounties and provisions are endless; it's cycle never ending.

So what happens when we make it dirty? When we contaminate our own water sources so completely that the water ceases to give life? What will happen then?

Water is spirit. Within us, encompassed in this secret of water exists a piece of the Divine. An element of God. When, through unclean practices we completely defile our spirit we fall spiritually ill. Without spiritual health you, as a healer cannot give health, spiritual or physical, to anyone. Your first line of defense is keeping your spirit clean and the source of your life giving gift will remain fluid, like water. Opposites attract. Your positive energy will attract negative energy and as a Hijama practitioner you need to know how to ground yourself from all the negative energy you absorb. Without a proper worship and meditation program, you will never last unless giving your sole over to darkness and using dark energy to then thrive. Hijama is good, healthy, light - cupping is the opposite.

**If you do not have a Sheikh, your Sheikh is Shatan!**

Those without an ijaaza will always become lost and eventually lose their way over to the dark side. No matter how much good intentions, no ijaaza means you are dedicated to serving Shatan, not Allah.

There is no gift like the gift of a healing, and no greater responsibility than to keep your own heart humble and free flowing with the water of the spirit that you are. When the water is pure, the heart is clear and the gift of healing flows easily through the healer. As water absorbs contamination from the environment around it, so does your spirit absorb the bad energy and dirtiness from those you treat and can cause illness of the soul and lead to spiritual illness and death. The windows of heaven are opening and many spiritually parched people smell the fresh water. The people are awakening to the existence of truly clean water again and they are going in search of it. As a healer and someone maintaining the sunnah of Hijama you are in a unique position to meet some of these individuals on their journey. Keeping your own spiritual health by daily meditation practices and a consistent routine to protect yourself from spiritually dark forces is an absolute requirement if you are to be prepared to really meet the needs of the people who come to you for Hijama. Along those lines, practicing Hijama without the authority and ijaaza to do so is going to become increasingly dangerous on a spiritual level. Those committing fraud by claiming to be practitioners without an ijaaza are headed for serious trouble both in this life and the hereafter.

A researcher from Japan named Masaru Emoto has literally performed hundreds of experiments to prove the effect of the energy resonated from the intention of a human being onto water. Using the control of exactly the same water source he placed water into jars and on the jars he wrote words. He wrote positive and negative words such as love and gratitude. He also played music in the presence of some bottles of water. Then he froze the water crystals and examined and photographed them. The absolutely most symmetrical and perfect circle with fine lines and well gathered clusters came from the water that was left in the presence of the reading of 'Holy Qur'an.'

The work from Dr. Emoto proves scientifically what holy (whole) people, saints or awliya have known all along, that words have profound power and spirituality and prayer are vitally important in altering health, society and the human soul. As Muslims we are instructed to begin everything with Besmillah ir rahman nir raheem- "In the name of Allah, the most merciful and most gracious." The energy resonance work performed by Dr. Emoto provides a better understanding as to why Allah (swt) instructed us to use these powerful words and phrases.

What Dr. Emoto's work does not touch upon is the corresponding need for the patient to believe all cures come from the Creator of All Things. This belief is not something obtained from making empty claims, it comes from obedience to the complete system Allah has provided for us to maintain this positive energy resonance throughout our lives. Through prayer, charity and thikr (remembrance or repeating of holy names) our acceptance of outside energy as well as creation of good energy within ourselves results in perfect health and existence within creation. A practitioner can impart good energy onto a patient, but if the patient does not continue a program of good living, they will return to poor health shortly after treatment. Most people want the quick fix and refuse to live in conformity with Gods orders that are designed to maximize benefits for us. Taking a pill, no matter the harm or adverse side effects is preferred by most foolish people.

Thikr Allah, literally meaning to remember God, it carries enormous healing benefits. We cannot possibly over emphasize the benefits of incorporating some sort of meditation practice into your daily routine. A discussion on the many benefits of meditation is beyond the scope of this current work, but we would encourage everyone to search out a program or meditation method most suited to each person and then practices it for at least one hour each day. Aspects of the energy resonance we discussed are vitally important as well as the breathing benefits that come from a dedicated meditation program. As stated before, all cures are from the Creator and connecting each day to the Creator is of paramount importance in leading a full, healthy and rich life. Our own choice of meditation practices are in our opinion the highest form of meditation available today, but any program that you prefer is better than nothing at all. You can read more about our recommended meditation practices at saltanat.org.

The mastery of Hijama, as a purely technical practice, can be easily obtained within hours of learning the practical elements of placing cups on optimal points of the body.

Anyone in this manner is easily able to perform Hijama on others. What we wish to stress here is the importance of the "energy resonance" a practitioner receives and imparts upon a patient as a key ingredient in becoming a qualified Hijama practitioner. This is not something that can be learned easily and is really a gift from Allah (swt).

Students should be invited to learn Hijama from a qualified and authorized master. Most students who are seeking to become a practitioner are running after a title and lack the humility and good character required to receive and impart good energy resonance. "I am doing this to revive the sunnah of Prophet Muhammad," is often the claim of people entering the field of Hijama. No, they are entering the field to be someone important and to make money. It is not wrong to accept money for services performed, but it must remain secondary to the process and yields far better results when it is a charity as opposed to a required payment. It may take a student ten or more years at the feet of a qualified master (sheikh) to develop the sensitivity to be able to receive and impart good energy or healing to a patient. Another student from their own life experience may be granted permission in a day.

Academic excellence has little to do with the ijaaza system of education. Certainly a student must be proficient in the technical aspects of a given discipline, but it is the spiritual advancement and maturity of the student that is being judged most. This is why the system of ijaaza is so important in protecting this ancient healing art form becoming a business practice performed by people who have no connection with a patient or understanding of how the spiritual life of the patient is profoundly married to their illness.

Clinical trials on pharmaceutical drugs always have to weigh the results of a placebo effect that the control sugar pill has in curing a person's ailment. Sixteen percent of all pharmaceutical drug trials that help people would have had the same positive effect from a sugar pill. When people pay (give charity) for a drug and believe it works, the outcome is positive even when there is no actual medicine prescribed.

We cannot stress enough the importance of finding a practitioner who is authorized – vetted by a true master and who does not claim on their own to have reached a level of understanding to truly receive and impart the energy necessary to effectuate positive healing and changes in patients' lives.

CHAPTER 7

## Glossary of Terms: Charity Blessings Saddaqa

# Understanding Charity and Healing

Today, there is much misunderstanding about charity and healing, which is why there is a need to educate people about these critically important concepts which are almost completely lost in the western world. Normally it would be considered self-serving, gauche, even embarrassing to openly discuss or raise these issues, however, the understanding is lost and therefore needs to be addressed.

Historically, the very act of talking about receiving charity, outside a framework of teaching, would decrease the spiritual power and blessings the charity brings; both for the person giving and for the person receiving the charity. It is said that charity is better given when the left hand does not know what the right hand is doing. Charity is better offered in secret. Seeking out those who are not asking for charity is preferred over those who are asking.

Healers who are asking for upfront payment, are little more than beggars. Healing and religion are not businesses. If they are focused on money, they are on the wrong way. It is that simple. We do not mean to be overly critical of those asking for upfront payments for services; there are plenty of well meaning people following what they understand to be the acceptable norms and methods for providing services. The proper understanding of healing and charity are almost lost - the client healer relationship suffers. Through education we hope to change that and restore age old values that actually worked to energize healing. It was recommended by an authorized teacher that if a patient would walk out of a session thinking they got away with cheating you, it is better today to charge the person for the service. We thus leave it to each authorized practitioner to follow their heart and always try to do what is best. As for the frauds, may Allah curse you for destroying the proper sunnah and respect for Prophet Muhammad (saw).

Money (a show of appreciation), historically, was offered to healers out of respect, not by demand. It was a good and honorable charity bringing with it an amount of protection and healing in and of itself. This is an age old understanding that has almost completely vanished from today's money driven corporate world. Inconspicuously, money, if that was what was given, was concealed in an envelope or small gift box and presented to the healer after the act of treatment - with full manners and respect and with an intention to provide a charitable reward, not payment.

The giving of charity is predominately for the protection and benefit of the giver. The healer, as with the holy (whole) person, normally one in the same, understands where his sustenance comes from and has no need to chase after it. When one becomes truly holy, sustenance chases after you.

Healers, as with holy persons, live simple lives. The money

that comes to them is for the benefit of mankind, not to enrich themselves. In this context, when given to the right person, charity heals mankind and heals the individual offering it. With correct charitable understanding giving the best one has to offer is ultimately benefits the giver as well as the society at large.

This action of giving charity actually boosts or empowers the overall effectiveness of the treatment. The treatment is a mechanism for the healing not the cause. Intention, respect, good manners and charity alters healing energy. The rewards from money well spent by someone spiritually higher than the giver, falls back on the giver. The closer the contribution is to something of real substance, such as gold, silver, or even a sheep, the more spiritual weight and protection that contribution of charity carries. Paper money, while acceptable, is less favorable. Checks and credit cards are negative in that the contribution is no longer inconspicuous.

Daily Charity Protects. As a standard course of protection for everyone, currently suffering from a spiritual, physical or mental illness or not, a box should be placed in their home for the purpose of contributing some measure of charity each day. The charity can be as small as a grain of rice, but should be commensurate with a person's means. Charity given once a day will provide much protection for an individual. Charity given twice a day will protect one's entire family from many things, seen and unseen; known and unknown. This is a major point to consider if good health and real happiness are the goal. Do not underestimate the power, protection and importance of giving charity. When the box starts to fill, listen to the heart and try to give the charity to someone who is in need but is not asking for charity. Nonetheless, try always to give some small amount of charity to anyone asking for it. One never knows who they might be in reality. Intention is everything.

The cure is not from the person through whom the healing comes. It certainly does do come from the treatment or even the charity.  The charity given is a contribution of thanks to the true healer, the Creator of all things. The person providing the service is entrusted with the charity - to use it in a wise and beneficial manner. It is not possible to pay enough for the gift of health. What is possible is to make certain that the intention is correct and pure and the offer is genuine. A grain of rice from a poor person can be much more genuine than a million dollars from a billionaire.

This is a rudimentary understanding of the benefits of charity and healing. It barely scratches the surface of the knowledge surrounding these issues. Charity's relationship to healing is profound and goes much deeper than we can imagine with our minds. Respect it, give it often and be happy for the gifts and benefits it brings. Follow Your Heart in all Matters.

CHAPTER 8

**Glossary of Terms:**
**Organic food Mineralization Local slow food Raw milk Nutrition value Halal meat Obesity Epidemic**

# A Comprehensive Cure

A brief overview of some of the problems brought on by our out of control technologically advanced society is in order. It should be understood that the eugenics movement mentioned earlier utilizes controls over the food chain to oppress and cull populations. Giving up control of our food and water supply and distribution chain to a few giant corporations has become a recipe for tyrannical rule over all people. Regulations "for your own safety" are being used to gain control over populations. Food has in fact become much less safe under industrialized farming techniques than the old local family farm to table system. Local natural food and raw milk producers are being forced out of business by regulations imposed on family farmers from lobbying efforts bought and paid for by the big agricultural industry. The UN Agenda 21 is at the root of this global assault on individual freedoms.

A Quick Look at the Dangers of Industrialized Farming

Following the Second World War corporations needed a market for their weapon making chemicals. The chemicals of nitrogen, potassium and phosphate were known to produce beautiful crops and these products which came to be known as NPK products were made readily available to farmers in the United States. The problem with these products was that while they worked to produce big beautiful vegetables, the vegetables were poor in nutritional value. The practice of NPK farming, along with the trend to grow one massive crop in the same field every year depleted the soil of valuable nutrition to the point that what we get on our supermarket shelves today are often referred to as "plastic veggies" by those who have learned the difference.

Many farmers came to understand the dangers of chemical fertilizers when their farm wells became irreversibly contaminated forcing many farms to fail and others to accept piped in fluoridated and chlorinated town water. For many it was too late to repair the damage to their fields and their water supply. For some, they moved to a more natural way of farming. Others got drug into the Monsanto nightmare of seeds which grow only one crop and are genetically modified leading to many more complications and resulting in a population that is getting sicker and sicker with each passing decade.

Industrial farmers have not found any solutions for these problems to date. The only solution is to return to a simplistic form of farming. Growing and eating locally produced food. Going back to the old ways of rotating crops and using the natural fertilization system of animal dung and other naturally occurring products in our local environments is the only hope we have of survival as a species. Any other direction will only lead us farther down the road to our own destruction. If you don't have a garden, plant one. If you have no place for a garden, move to a place where you can plant one!

### A Word about Organic Foods

Expensive and the best choice when forced to purchase store bought foods, organic fruits and vegetables can still leave your body lacking what it needs for good health. These foods are often shipped from China, Mexico etc and, while better than nonorganic, are still tremendously deficient in nutrients and medicinal value. Just because it says organic does not mean that the soils that grow the food have the mineral content necessary to keep your body healthy and strong and with long distance travel time organic foods quickly loose vitamin and mineral content. It is imperative that practitioners educate their patients about the importance of taking effective and naturally produced vitamin and mineral supplements to provide proper nutrition.

The obesity epidemic in the world is primarily a function of low nutrients in the food supply. Our brains tell us to keep eating even though we have consumed more calories than we should be consuming. If your body receives the right nutrients, you eat much less food and feel satisfied. Of course GMO foods, high fructose corn syrup and other major artificial substances in the food supply contribute to the obesity epidemic as well.

What we want to emphasize here is that real vegetables have levels of flavorful nutrition. Once you switch to eating organically home grown fruits and vegetables you will begin to feel the energy that your body has been missing. You will even find that you crave the wonderful flavors found in your own garden and will feel so much more satisfied after consuming a small salad than you ever felt was possible.

**Real Halal Meat Products**

Industrialized meat processing plants that produce the hamburger you purchase in the plastic wraps sold in many big box grocery stores are estimated to contain meat from over one-thousand different cows. The chances of a person contracting food borne illness greatly increase in these industrialized meat processing facilities. To combat these many problems the industry sprays the meat with various bacteria designed to combat other more dangerous bacteria on the meat products. To increase productivity and output cows are feed all sorts of growth hormones and chemicals designed to make cows grow faster and yield more meat. Antibiotics are used to counter the many diseases that occur from keeping so many cows in small areas while waiting to be slaughtered. All in all, this is not a good recipe for producing real halal meat. Don't eat it! Work to develop halal meat processing with others in your community. Find one member who has a farm and support their efforts to grow good clean meat for all of the community.

While most Muslims believe they understand how to properly slaughter an animal most efforts fall short of the requirements for real halal processing. Among many other requirements, animals must be treated gently, with great respect, calmed down, segregated from other living animals for the actual slaughter and given a drink of water just before slaughtering. When performed properly a peace descends upon the process that should be evident to all who witness the slaughtering. We truly are what we eat.

There is a growing movement in America to buy slow local food. Slow local food will provide you and your family with greater nutrition and even medicinal value, as good clean food is medicine. GMO food products are literally poison foods and should be entirely outlawed, but as long as money can buy congress the industry headed by Monsanto will continue to prevail. Today most food products in the major grocery stores are slow kill weapons. Once you begin this journey and really begin to understand what good nutritional and clean food is, you will find that 90% of the food on supermarket shelves falls into the poison category.

**The Simple Life**

Generally, going to bed with the sun and rising before sunrise is the healthiest practice. The property of electricity, while offering some convenience and benefit, has done more harm than good for mankind. Learning to live without it can be an exhilarating and freeing experience. You can never know what true silence is until you have sat in the mountains, or the wilderness where there are no electrical power lines and no buzzing of appliances. The silence is golden. Your thikr is stronger. Your connection to the real world, much clearer. When Imam Al Mehdi (as) returns it is mentioned by awliya that three takbeers will be sounded at a critical time where mankind is on the brink of total destruction. At that point the very property of electricity will cease to exist. This will have an immediate and profound effect on mankind and society in turning us back into real human beings. People are free to believe or not believe such things, but what we should understand now is that a simple life and simple society is always best. To the extent that people can simplify their lives, make them more natural, keep away from processed and artificial things, the healthier they will become.

CHAPTER 9

## Glossary of Terms:
## Wusil Wudu Niat Attar
## Cardiovascular system

# Belief and the Physical Response

Today, everyone believes they can become an expert from books and on-line courses. When we are speaking of Hijama, and any other type of healing treatment, whether traditional or alternative, academics are secondary to actual healing energy and power. The power to effect healing is a gift, not a certificate to be bought.

Hijama is a religious practice, as is circumcision. Actually, all healing arts are religiously based practices as all healing comes from the Creator. Hijama should be performed by someone who has apprenticed under an authorized person. It is not a business and any amount of licensing and control will only degrade the benefits of Hijama as both a physically and spiritually holistic and charitable practice.

By healers, we mean individuals "authorized" by real masters who focus on the spiritual, physical and mental well-being of the human being seeking assistance. Morality and spiritual enlightenment are of paramount importance in considering whom to authorize with this honored trust. Not solely mental capacity or technical ability.

As long as the Hijama Master is alive, students of this art are sent to the Master to be authorized. Authorization is not simply asserting technical proficiency. It is something much higher - way beyond a person's mental capacity. These concepts and teachings can only be understood in the heart - in the realm of spiritual knowledge. They must be sanctioned and activated by someone who has successfully achieved these understandings from their Master. Claiming to be a Master does not make it so. The mind cannot decipher between a real Master and a fraud. Certainty comes only when the heart judges, not the mind. A healer is raised, provided with a gift to heal, not trained.

The recent work by Masuru Emoto, discussed in an earlier chapter, on energy resonance provides a scientific basis for this otherwise spiritual understanding. Energy resonance changes matter and alters the physical property of cells. The more spiritually enlightened a person is, the stronger this energy and the better the result. This is true in all healing professions. As much as someone can place positive energy on a patient, they can also do harm. The very process of entering into a patient/healer relationship authorizes the transfer of energy. With this in mind, it is very important to consider just who you allow to put their hands on you, especially for the purpose of treating your body for illness related problems. People put off energy. The only consideration is whether that energy is positive or negative. Women permitting male doctors to interfere in the birthing process are harming themselves and their babies. All contact with men and pregnancy is negative. Angels are assigned to a developing child in the womb and should be left alone as much as possible. Midwives are the best practitioners when it comes to giving birth. Ultrasound is doing so much harm to the unborn fetus and never should be performed. Good to note here,

The practical aspects of Hijama are quite simple; the healing aspects are much more complex and should not come from a practitioner who has chosen for themselves to become a "health care provider". Masters recognize a student that shows promise, and then cultivate and nurture that natural God given ability and then give permission to practice when the student is spiritually, physically and mentally prepared. In fact permission only comes from Muhammad (saw).

People saying otherwise are the same people saying anyone can be a scholar and anyone can be a leader. Foolishness! You are not elected - you are selected. But our egos are saying, "No, I can do whatever I want; I am smarter than he/she is and better fit for that job." This is the ego's incorrect and arrogant thinking. Today everyone is a king or queen of their own domain. They research a subject or discipline on the Internet and suddenly they are experts. No one wants to be a common servant, but servanthood is one of the doorways to heaven and one that will bring with it so much blessing!

True Hijama is only performed by authorized persons given permission by other authorized persons with a chain of authorization back to Prophet Muhammad (saws). You will hear that often from us. Not to promote ourselves, but to make people understand that learning what follows does not qualify someone to perform Hijama. Many people from many walks of life and ways of thinking are performing cupping, but this is not Hijama. If you are a cupper and a

Muslim, do not delude yourself into thinking that you are fulfilling the Sunnah of Rasool'allah simply by performing the physical act of cupping. Without permission, you are degrading the Sunnah and making a mockery of it because without the spiritual nature that comes with properly performing Hijama the power of healing is absent.

Real healers are servants unto their Lord Almighty, full stop. Ask yourselves what is the difference between a real holy person who can guide you along your spiritual path and a psychic or fortuneteller? These are important questions and distinctions that people need to understand to avoid the traps of Shatan (Satan) and keep from falling into false concepts and ideas. The ijaaza system is intended to safeguard against these fraudulent agents of evil who come claiming to be able to heal you and help you determine your future. Without the ijaaza system anyone can claim knowledge and understanding and corrupt the ancient healing methods that have worked for centuries to help cure people of illnesses effecting the mind, body and spirit.

**Benefits of Hijama - Why it Works**

Because God sanctioned it as a cure, full stop!

That said . . . .

The cardiovascular system is made up of the heart and all of the blood and lymphatic vessels in the body. The heart acts as a pump to drive the blood; a complex fluid made up of digested food materials, respiratory gasses (oxygen being carried in, carbon dioxide being carried out), and protective and regulatory chemicals through the approximately 60,000 miles of vessels in the body.

More than 90 percent of Americans live in jeopardy of having a serious illness related to the circulatory system. The human and financial cost of cardiovascular disease in the U.S. alone is astronomical. Every year, approximately 1.5 million Americans have a heart attack, 300,000 of whom die before receiving medical attention.

Hijama does not heal your body or have a direct effect on immediate medical problems; per se. Hijama cleans the body's cardiovascular system so disease never has a chance to develop. Where disease already exists, Hijama cleans the system to help the body better fight and recover from the disease. Noticeable benefits from Hijama often come weeks, even months after a Hijama session. It is very foolish to wait until the point that your body is showing signs of illness.

Hijama is best utilized as a preventative maintenance procedure for your body. In short, it better enables your body to heal itself -- No drugs, no expensive treatment or therapy and above all, no operations.

Hijama removes dead blood cells from the cardiovascular system. It is a bit like getting your radiator flushed. It should be done before your car overheats and the damage to your engine block or hoses is done. Practitioners who emphasize Hijama and cupping as a quick cure for serious acute and/or chronic illnesses are like auto mechanics who claim flushing your radiator will cure your cracked engine block. Of course, your radiator should be flushed, but if it were properly maintained no damage would have resulted to your engine in the first place. Fortunately, the body, unlike an engine block, can often repair itself because our bodies are made of rejuvenating cells. It is because of this attribute of the human body that Hijama can be called a cure for all illness because while not eliminating the chronic or acute illness immediately, the procedure will promote rejuvenation and this will lead to the cure you seek. In the case of some ailments and conditions, such as heart failure and stroke, hijama can have a very positive effect if applied as soon after the event as possible. However, it is always better to use Hijama as a maintenance and preventative procedure.

CHAPTER 10

**Glossary of Terms: Blood clotting Moderate exercise Menopause Menses Acupuncture points Meridian Acupressure message Lymphatic system**

# Practical Application of Hijama

### Who should have Hijama?

Hijama is predominately prescribed for sexually active men thirty and older. Women are less susceptible to problems associated with cardiovascular illness until they reach the age of menopause. The monthly discharge of blood has a somewhat similar effect as Hijama. When a woman's monthly course stops, preventative Hijama should be instituted as an annual or biannual preventative procedure for women. If special problems exist, Hijama may be performed on women before menopause, but not during menses or pregnancy.

Hijama is an excellent remedy for persons with hypertension (high blood pressure). Those suffering from high blood pressure should be routinely cupped in the spring and fall until pressure normalizes. Proceed thereafter once a year as a preventative maintenance. In cases where high blood pressure results from abnormal cell growth from lifelong exposure to toxic chemical or directly related to kidney dysfunction, Hijama is less effective but still helps. In these cases drastic lifestyle changes are normally required to see significant improvement.

Abnormal blood cells are not dead and Hijama will not remove abnormal cells until they die. Perform Hijama to optimizing your system and combat the effects of abnormal cell growth caused by environmental exposures. Environmental illness normally requires a complete change in lifestyle to a naturally organic diet with regular exercise. Hijama healers should educate themselves on these very real and modern illnesses which are increasing in the world population at an exponential rate.

While Hijama can be an effective treatment for many emergency care situations a discussion of the use of Hijama in emergency medicine is beyond the scope of this current work. It has been reported by Prophet Muhammad (saws) as being a cure for all illnesses. We do not dispute this. As mentioned earlier, conditions such as modern environmental exposure, toxicity, etc. are more like a limb being cut off than an illness. Hijama will not make you grow a new arm or attach a severed leg. If you surgically can reattach the limb, Hijama will certainly help it heal faster. Environmental illnesses require drastic lifestyle changes.

Once again, we remind you that this information is intended for educational purposes, not as a substitute for proper training by a qualified Hijama Master.

Persons should also contact their doctors and not rely upon Hijama as a substitute for standard medical care. (Legal Disclaimer)

## Preparing and Cleanliness

Both the patient and the practitioner should be clean, physically and spiritually, for the Hijama process by taking a shower with the intention of physical and spiritual protection and cleanliness. In Arabic and among Muslims this is known as Wusil or Wudu. In English these terms translate as ablution. After the shower, apply natural perfume oils, called ittar (attar) in the Arabic tongue, that attract angelic beings and also have medicinal benefits. You may chose pure rose, bakoor or a botanical musk or oud. Place some on your wrist before starting the Hijama procedure. These oils should always be worn for the spiritual benefits they offer. They also smell fantastic. Real perfume oils are chemical free and almost always non-allergenic as the pollen which causes natural allergies is not present in the oils extracted from plants.

Always make a dua (prayer) before beginning and always begin each action with bismilla ir rahman ir rahim. This translates as "In the name of God, Most Gracious, Most Merciful." Offer two rakas (prostrations) of thanks for the healing you are about to receive. Make the intention to fulfill the sunnah of Prophet Muhammad (saws). Hijama should be performed in the seated position facing the Qibla unless medical circumstances do not permit.

The practical application of Hijama that we offer can easily be described as the most conservative approach to Hijama. The techniques incorporated into this spiritual practice of the Sunnah are based on a very old healing art sanctioned by Prophets and utilized by healers over the centuries.

Most of you will unfortunately ignore our warnings about finding a qualified Hijama practitioner with an authorized ijaaza to perform Hijama. This is most unfortunate as it degrades Islam on the whole and permits the enemies of Islam to further belittle Islamic practices. From a purely technical standpoint, if patients adhere to one steadfast rule they should be able to avoid the dangers associated with the incorrect and overuse of cupping therapy. The first and foremost rule is never sleep after Hijama. Moderate exercise on the day of Hijama or cupping is most important. The risk of blood clotting is real although very rare! Patients should stay awake. This is one of the primary reasons why Hijama is performed in the morning. Take a brisk walk after the procedure is performed. If it is cold outside, walk indoors and stay warm. There is a tendency to want to sleep, but this must be avoided. We cannot emphasis this enough. People who are saying otherwise are putting you at risk and may be causing more problems than they are solving.

While there are certain dangers in doing Hijama on the wrong days and we encourage people to abide by the lunar odd day requirements; if performed on the wrong days it will simply result in no real benefits obtained. Some of the prophetic sayings warn against certain days, especially Wednesdays and many spiritual masters teach that cutting hair or letting blood on Saturday is disrespectful of the Jewish Sabbath and so should be avoided. Optimal days are the odd days falling on Monday, Tuesday or Thursday.

Practitioners espousing the need for multiple consecutive sessions over days or weeks are doing so generally to make more money. It is sufficient to do Hijama twice a year, no more. Doing more, when done properly will likely have no adverse effects. For chronic conditions there may be some benefits. Patients need to decide for themselves. We recommend no more than twice a year.

**Optimal Points for Hijama**

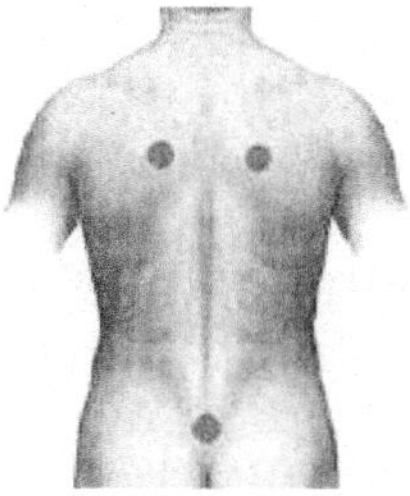

As stated earlier, Hijama is very conservative compared to the modern day therapy called cupping. The traditional points for Hijama to rid the entire body of dead blood cells when performed in the same session are;

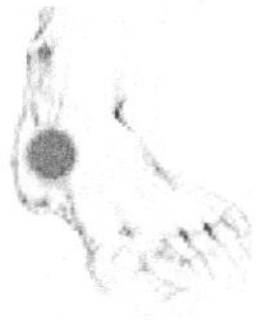

1. The two points adjacent to the seventh vertebra (heart position in acupuncture terms) on the back, approximately two inches from the spine.
2. The tail of the spine

3. The two inner positions of the feet on the

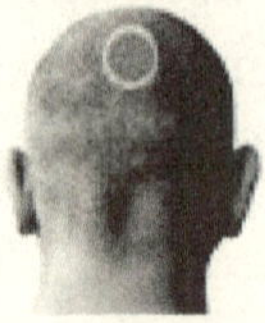

ankle (great care should be take here).

4. The top back side of the head normally where balding first starts and the hair moves out from all directions.

When the above points are performed in one session it is sufficient to clean the entire body. No other points on the body need to be performed when all of these points are performed during the same Hijama session. Most patients will not accept Hijama on the back of the head as shaving the spot that needs to be cupped is unacceptable to most patients. However, it is highly recommended that all these points be performed in one session to clean the entire body.

We only recommend Hijama on the head on the 19th and 21st days of the lunar month corresponding to Monday, Tuesday and Thursdays.

These above described locations are the only Hijama positions that we advise for preventative Hijama and the positions we cup ourselves. Excessive use of Hijama is unnecessary and can be harmful. All patients should be provided Hijama in the sitting position unless medical circumstances don't allow it.

For specific complaints and local injury, Hijama can be applied most anywhere that it is possible to place a cup and obtain a good seal. Hijama practitioners should exercise good judgment when applying cups to sensitive areas of the body. Most cupping practitioners have taken to charging per cup and thus the economic pressures to over cup are very real - a practice we strongly discourage.

However, if properly performed, overuse of cupping will likely have no real adverse impact on one's health. Nonetheless, conservative Hijama practices are recommended because infection and the potential marks resulting from Hijama are possible. It is normally sufficient to use one cup to alleviate local conditions or injury and for one session only.

There are varying opinions about the best places to place the cups. Acupuncture points may or may not provide insight into the best positions to cup. Common sense suggests that there is some correlation but evidence is almost all anecdotal. Some mention of optimal places to cup is made in the sayings or teachings of Prophet Muhammad (saws). The strength or accuracy of some of these teachings is sometimes debated amongst the scholars. These above concerns and points of debate mostly boil down to arguments that frustrate the practice and cause unnecessary concerns for patients.

True healers listen to the patient and then combine that information with a sense where the injury is present. It is a process of training that requires the practitioner to listen to their heart not their mind and know from spiritual understanding what place on the body will result in the most benefit from Hijama. This is not something you can learn in books. Those persons trained in Reiki and polarity will likely have a better idea what we are attempting to convey here.

## Hijama Supplies

Previously washed and stored **cups** should be boiled or run through a hot dishwasher the night before the procedure is to be performed. Following the procedure cups can be cleaned in a 1:4 bleach solution and then sterilized before storing.

The shape or architecture of professional cups normally does provide a better bond and greater suction but a simple baby food jar will do in a pinch. Suction cups eliminate the need for fire. We generally do not recommend using a pump system or vacuum cups. While there may be no real harm, the benefits will likely be diminished. The element of fire likely has benefits not fully understood. Providing some sterility is just one known benefit. Regulating the amount of pull or suction so one does not create too much suction on the body is another possible benefit. Practitioners should always respect the prescribed methods and adhere to them as best as possible. That said, we do have to admit to utilizing the suction tools on occasion. If you do use the suction cups be very careful not to apply too much pressure to the skin.

**Kerosene** is a far better choice for cleaning the skin after treatment than alcohol. You can dip your paper cones in it for better ignition when using the fire element. The higher the grade of kerosene the better. Most store bought brands for indoor lamps are not suitable as they contain dies. The best source is usually a paint store where they sell pure kerosene.

A normal store bought **candle** is perfect for Hijama. The candle is lit and placed on a table next to the person being cupped. By utilizing a candle it reduces the need for individually lighting each paper cone with a match or lighter. The practitioner needs to have both hands free to perform Hijama properly. Candles provide the flexibility and freedom to light the cones quickly and apply them before the cup becomes too hot and burns the patient. With a little practice, burning is rare. Don't forget **matches** to light the candle!

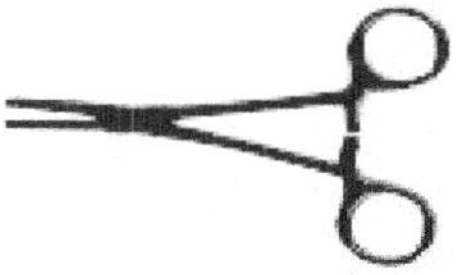

**Cotton balls** work well but cost money. It is always cheaper and often times more effective to use small **paper cones** made from old newspaper, especially if using the traditional fire technique. The kerosene and fire are sufficient to sterilize the paper and poses no health hazard.

A **hemostat** is a surgical instrument designed to pinch veins or arteries when operating on a patient. Most medical supply stores can provide you with them. Some places are reluctant to sell them as they are often used as roach clips (something used to hold the end of the marijuana cigarette). As a result you can find them in most "head shops". Long tweezers will work also but present an additional danger of dropping a flaming paper cone or cotton ball on the carpet or worse yet a patient.

Most any store that carries paint supplies will have

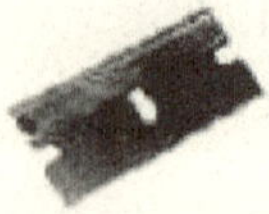

**single edge razor blades**. They are very cheap and disposable and you must use a **new razor blade on each patient**. Razors are soaked in a dish of kerosene before using them to make the small incisions. This reduces the risk of infection in the skin following the procedure.

A box of **regular, unscented, store bought**

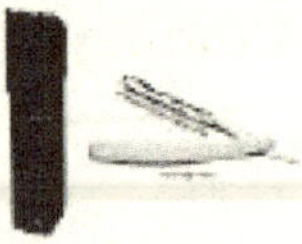

**tissue** is necessary for catching blood while removing the cups as well as for general cleanup. **Non latex surgical gloves** should be worn to protect you from the blood of the patient and the patient from any open sores on your hands.

When performing Hijama on areas covered with hair, **clippers** to remove longer hair and **shaving supplies** to remove short hair and better provide a clean smooth surface for the cups to adhere, is necessary. Men will often require their backs to be shaved in the areas where Hijama will be performed; otherwise cups will lose suction and fall off.

A **sturdy high table** is needed to provide easy access and a workable surface for Hijama supplies. A **message chair** or a **simple kitchen chair turned backwards** is sufficient for the patient. A **garbage can** for the used tissue, blood and paper cones and a **small tub** for used cups.

A light breakfast should be offered to patients after Hijama as fasting before is a requirement. Patients should eat a small amount and then walk for one half to one hour.

### Instructions and Facts to Discuss with the Patient

- Persons interested in Hijama need to abstain from sexual intercourse 48 hours before the treatment is scheduled.

- The day of the procedure patients should avoid food and drink nine hours before the procedure, especially dairy products. One cup of Non-acidic herbal tea is permitted to help waken.

- A warm shower should be taken as close to the time of the procedure as practical.

- The tendency to become tired after Hijama and want to rest is common but resting must be avoided for at least the first few hours after the procedure. This is why we schedule all Hijama sessions in the morning to avoid people from resting soon after the procedure and to make the fasting easier. Inactivity can result in the promotion of blood clotting, which is why resting is highly discouraged. In fact a half hour to one hour walk is highly recommended. The danger of clotting is rare but nonetheless possible, especially if falling asleep after the procedure.

- Red marks from the hijama normally fade within a few days, depending on skin type. Do not scratch the Hijama areas.

- The small shallow incisions necessary to extract the dead blood cells may take a few weeks to heal. In some cases faint tiny lines of scarring may persist.

## Getting Started

As directed previously, Hijama is best performed in the morning to enable people to fast before the procedure and to facilitate and ensure that patients remain active and do not rest or sleep following their Hijama procedure.

Depending upon the number of people being given Hijama you should select an area with plenty of space. One area designated as a waiting room, a more private area for the actual hijama, and a separate place to take a quick bite to eat following the procedure. We normally offer people some sort of small healthy breakfast with juice and tea. Our actual Hijama area is often set up in a garden area being careful to make sure the patients do not get cold. Cooler days, you should move the operation indoors. It is very important to have a good workable area to perform the Hijama.

A table with all Hijama supplies and equipment set up adjacent to the chairs where the patients will sit is very important to facilitate the quick and efficient removing and replacing of cups.

An experienced Hijama practitioner can work on several patients at one time. A competent assistant must be present standing in front of the chairs and patients, looking for any signs of fainting. Ideally you also want an assistant standing next to you to clean used cups and help with other necessary chores. With proper planning it is possible to facilitate a hundred or more patients in one given day. With such limited ideal days for preventative Hijama, five days in the spring and five days in the fall, the attendance is often very high.

The direction of the chairs should face towards the southeast when performing Hijama in most southern states in the USA. These are spiritual matters that will not be understood with simple explanations. These are some of the subjects more deeply discussed when trained by a true master. Other spiritual oddities and concerns are discussed or rather introduced below. We are not anticipating your blind acceptance, but as there is no obvious harm in doing these things, better safe than sorry.

As an experiment take a tesbih (a string of beads used for thikr - counting Divine names) hold them by the top part of the string. Rotate the beads in a circular motion, counter clockwise, until they make a smooth circle. Hold your hand very still and wait until the beads begin to move in a diagonal direction back and forth. The direction for facing while being given Hijama is in one of the two directions that the beads will swing. One of those two directions corresponds with the direction that Muslims pray towards the Kabbah. If you want an explanation as to why this works, you must ask someone who really knows. There are not many, but if you look, you will find.

Chairs are actually placed in the reverse position so that patients may straddle the back and have something to lean on if they start to feel weak. A common sturdy wooden kitchen chair with a proper back is often best.

### Hemostat Method

With hemostat clipped to a cotton ball in one hand and a cup in the other dominate hand (open side facing down), dip the cotton ball into the kerosene and gently shake off the excess kerosene before placing it in the candle's flame to ignite the cotton ball. You never want the cotton ball to be soaked thus dripping little fire balls all over; the ground, patient or your assistant. Quickly move the burning cotton ball underneath the open end of the cup and insert the burning cotton ball towards the back or bottom of the cup. Timing is everything here and practice will make you an expert. Too much burning time in the cup, and you may burn yourself. You also run the risk of branding your patient. With practice burning is rare. Take the burning cotton ball out too quickly, and the suction will not be sufficient to have the desired effect.

In one smooth and continuous quick motion remove the burning cotton ball from the cup and position the cup on the prescribed spot. Deliberately push the cup into the skin making certain that you form a strong seal. Gently remove your grip to see if you achieved a good seal. You should be able to flick the cup with your finger without any possibility of the cup falling off. You may also try to wiggle the cup back and forth to test the seal. If you achieved a good seal with proper suction, the skin will begin to puff up in a few seconds. If the seal is weak, remove the cup and start over. You must have a good seal and proper suction.

### Cone Method

Take ordinary notebook paper or newspaper and tear them into inch and a half square pieces. You will need to make a minimum of three cones for each individual Hijama procedure (three square pieces of paper).

It is much better to make plenty of cones so you are certain not to run out at a critical point Wrap the paper around your index finger and twist the pointed end at the bottom of the cone.

Pay close attention to the length of the cone as it must easily fit into the cup. To shorten the cone you may fold back part of the twisted end.

The twisted end will act as the handle to hold the cone with the flared end of the cone being dipped into the kerosene and then ignited with the candle flame. Once you have ignited the cone you tilt the cup in one hand on its side and toss the burning cone into the bottom of the cup, quickly placing the cup on the desired position.

The cone method is much easier to master than the hemostat method. Because the paper remains burning in the cup, the suction created by the increased heat is almost always more efficient than the hemostat method. The added burning time also promotes greater sterilization. The burning paper will quickly go out after the cup is applied to the skin. In some cases the paper may cause some burning if falling back against the skin. This is normally very minor. With the cone method it is common for the cup to fill with smoke. The smoke will not block your ability to see the blood in the cup.

**Suction Cup Method**

There are several new kits on the market that provide a suction method for extracting the air from the cups placed on a patient. The quality and effectiveness of the kits vary greatly. One of the primary concerns is cups will deform when placed in a conventional dishwasher. These kits should be avoided at all cost as it is near impossible to effectively sterilize the cups between uses. Some people dispose of the cups, using them only once, which is an option you may use if you do not mind the added costs. There are plastic cups that are dishwasher safe and can be adequately sterilized and cleaned for further use. You must make certain your dishwasher is set to a temperature that will kill all possible pathogens. There is only one glass Hijama set on the market that we are currently aware of and sell on our website. This kit is much higher quality than most others that we have seen.

In general we favor the conventional fire method. The potential to create too much suction by over pumping the cups is one primary cause of concern. Additionally, we believe that the actual property of fire has benefits not fully understood, as well as providing some additional sterility. Lastly, the small openings where the suction pump is placed can be areas where pathogens accumulate and are more difficult to sterilize.

The benefits of using the suction pump method include eliminating the chances of burning the skin and ease of use. Most practitioners will opt to offer their patients a choice after explaining the differences.

Continuing Hijama...

Now leave the cup on and proceed to the next spot to be cupped.

Each initial cup will normally take about five to fifteen minutes. The area will develop a pinkish red hickey mark. Once this color becomes pinkish red you are ready for the second step.

Removing cups...

Cups are best removed by holding your thumb on one section near the rim of the cup. Gently push down with your thumb and tilt back the cup away from the thumb pressure point. You will start to hear the air escape from the cup. In fact, the air is rushing into the cup.

Once the cup is removed, a quarter inch or more raised pinkish red welt with no blistering or burns is the desired result. Blistering and burns means too much heat and possibly having left the cup on longer than required. You may still proceed with apparent burns and blisters but the pain and healing process will be prolonged.

Remove the new single edge razor from the kerosene where it has been soaking for sterilization purposes.

Make seven tiny incisions into the pinkish red circle on the skin. These incisions do not have to be very long. 1/16 to 1/8 of an inch is sufficient. Try to keep the incisions away from the edge of the red welted circle. More than an actual cutting motion, the desired movement should be a controlled jab making certain not to penetrate the skin too deeply. Never attempt this until you have practiced on an orange. Most orange skins resemble the resistance and properties of human skin. You can slice the skin off the orange to test your depth. Your goal is to just penetrate the derma, not to go deep into any tissue under the skin. The pressure is not more than tapping your finger or a car key against a glass window without any fear of breaking it

Once you have made the tiny incisions, you must quickly heat the interior of the cup and replace it on the exact same spot. As soon as you have placed a properly sealed cup on the area, dead blood cells already brought to the surface by the first hijama procedure will almost immediately start to be drawn from the patient.

If the suction is not sufficient and a proper seal achieved you may have to wipe the blood from the area before attempting to replace the cup. The blood will disrupt the new seal.

If the cup fills rather quickly, it is best to remove the cup, empty out the blood, and repeat the procedure again. Twice is usually sufficient to remove all the dead blood cells. It is normal for someone who has never had Hijama to release more blood than those who have been given Hijama before.

When performing Hijama on the back shoulder and head, have the patient gently move their arms, hands and fingers. It is advisable to also gently stretch one's neck from side to side, being careful not to dislodge the cups.

A great benefit for the eyes is to take clean water and splash the water into the eyes while the cup is on the head and is removing blood. This was recommended by the Prophets and

Saints as a means for curing eye problems. The patient should sat, "In the Name of God" while splashing the water into the eyes. In the heavenly language, “Bismillah ir Rahman nir Raheem.”

All blood products are best buried in the ground as it is part of your living being. It is also not good to let the blood be available to people who have knowledge of the occult and beings in the unseen worlds. This again is a subject beyond the scope of this work. What we recommend is a protection for you, accept it. Flushing it down the toilet into a septic system may suffice as a burial method.

After removing the final cup, immediately wipe the area clean with a tissue soaked in kerosene. Kerosene is by far the best solution to use as it disinfects, stops any additional bleeding, and promotes rapid healing of the wound. It works much better than alcohol.

The kerosene should have been sufficient to stop any additional bleeding. To be safe, place a dry tissue over the area to keep any stains off of clothing. No need to bandage the area as exposure to the air is beneficial. Patients should refrain from showering for one day and not scrub the area for several days. Some itching is expected and scratching should be avoided as it will contribute to scaring.

To receive optimal health benefits, patients should take a walk for one half hour or more to keep the circulation moving. If food is being served, (highly recommended) eat only a small healthy breakfast, preferably no coffee or heavy foods.

It is quiet normal for patients to report feeling light and energized days and weeks after the procedure. The curative effects of Hijama will continue months after the procedure. Many chronic conditions will slowly begin to disappear over the days, weeks and months to follow.

Begin your experience by thanking God, by saying; "In God's name we begin". Dedicate the healing procedure (Hijama) for the honor of the most honored amongst mankind, Prophet Muhammad (saws) - this brings much more power. End the experience by giving charity in thanks. Have full respect and good manners when partaking of the benefits provided to you by your Creator.

## Hygiene

The level of hygiene you incorporate into the Hijama session is frankly a decision you must follow according to your own situation and understanding. There are practitioners who have been performing Hijama for decades and have never used gloves or have any concern with blood borne illnesses. They have never contracted a single illness. I share this with you so that you may reflect on the level of spiritual understanding and trust which they posses. Never would I recommend anyone to not incorporate a high level of hygiene into their Hijama practice, but it is worth mentioning. In the West, patients have grown to expect a high level of hygiene.

Regardless of the level of protection you decide for yourself, it is recommended that you trust God, but also tie your horse. All cups and equipment should be soaked in a solution of 1:4 bleach solutions before being used in any Hijama procedure and most dishwashers provide hot water sufficient to sterilize cups and equipment.

Cups should never be used on another patient unless thoroughly sterilized. Our advice in using bleach may or may not be sufficient or a standard that is acceptable to kill all pathogens. Hydrogen peroxide may be better, heat is preferred. All persons already engaged in Hijama and incorporating what we offer here in the way of advice should use their own judgment and knowledge in providing sterile and safe environments for their patients.

CHAPTER 11

**Glossary of Terms:**
**Lunar calendar Tidal influence**
**Islamic calendar Full moon Odd lunar days**

# Understanding Tidal Influences

## Lunar Forces & Effects on the Body

Just as the moon affects the tide of the ocean, it affects the human body. Therefore, Hijama should be performed on odd days of the lunar calendar when the forces of the moons pull assist in removing the dead blood cells. It is important to note that most practitioners blindly adhere to the commonly accepted Islamic calendar dates established in Saudi Arabia. These calendar dates are based on local moon sightings and can often times be in contradiction with the actual odd day. For example, if it is cloudy one day and the moon cannot be sighted it is sunnah (Prophetic tradition) to wait till the moon can be sighted. If conditions continue to not permit sighting then the new month automatically starts after the 30th day of the previous months sighting. This is fine to keep the community fasting and praying on the same days, but it does nothing to accurately determine the odd day as it relates to tidal forces. It is the tidal forces pulling out the blood from the body like water from the shore, which is of paramount importance. The good news is that if you get it wrong there will be no harm, but clients will not receive optimum results. Once practitioners establish an authentic odd date, they should continue to calculate the odd dates from that confirmed date.

It should also be done in the second half of the lunar month. The 17th, 19th, and 21st days are the best for hijama. While less favorable, Hijama can also be performed on the 23rd and 25th days of the lunar month. You may utilize the full moon (15th) and tidal charts to help determine the lunar odd days.

Moderate climate is also important, not to hot and not to cold. When the flowers start to blossom and nature begins its magical renewal, it is time for Hijama. Hijama may also be performed in the early fall, before the first frost.

You may have heard that the tide comes in and the tide goes out, but in fact a tide is the vertical movement of water and only goes up and down. Current is the horizontal or sideways flow of water. The current floods which make the tide rise and ebb out and make the tide fall. A tide is the rise and fall of water caused by gravitational forces of the moon and sun on the oceans of the earth.

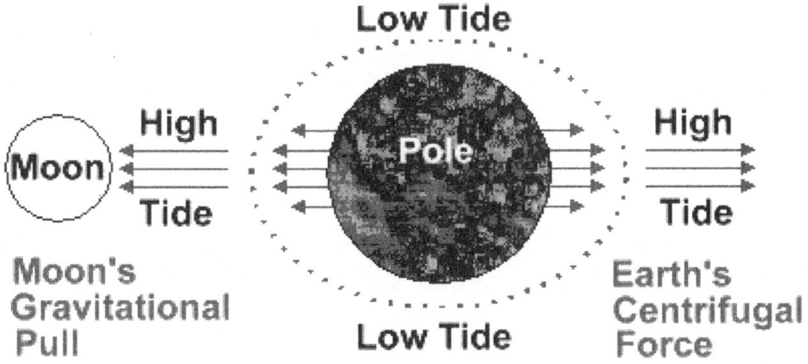


How do the movements of the sun and the moon affect tide? The gravitational pull of the moon tugs on the surface of the ocean until its surface mounds up and outward in the direction of the moon. When the mound of water has reached its highest point it is called high tide. On the opposite side of the earth from the moon, the centrifugal force caused by the earth's rotation produces another mound of water and high tide. Between these two high tides are two flat areas on the surface of the ocean which are the low tides.

Each day there are two high tides and two low tides. The time between high and low tide is a little over 6 hours and the entire tidal cycle repeats itself four times each day. The regularity of the tides corresponds to the regular orbit of the moon around the earth and the rotation of the earth as it orbits around the sun.

Depending upon the position of the moon relative to the earth and sun, a moon can have different phases. The phases of the moon are also very regular, and have been used for thousands of years to keep track of time using the lunar calendar. In addition to the daily movements of the moon, these monthly lunar cycles can also impact the tides.

CHAPTER 12

# Final Considerations

Hijama is a procedure instituted by Prophets and Saints who possess a spiritual understanding of healing far beyond what scientists and contemporary medical doctors understand. Spiritual men understand that all cures are from God and the plant, herb, knowledge or procedure is just the catalyst for the cure originating from above. The catalyst is favored and improved by proper respect and manners. A procedure done with the intention of reviving the ways of the Prophets and Saints carries much more power and benefit with it - an understanding almost completely lost today.

Healing is an order that comes from God. It is facilitated by both healers and angels who are ordered to partake in the process of the healing. All healing is a miracle. Never say that the Hijama healed me or the herb healed me or the healer healed me. No, only God heals.

When properly attributed to God the healing takes a power it otherwise would not have. It is assisted by angels who are working with the process. As in the case of Hijama, angels are helping to push out the dead blood cells from the body and scrubbing the thousands of miles of arteries, veins and capillaries that the human body contains. Analysis of extracted blood from Hijama shows that only dead blood cells are removed. How is this possible - no living blood cells coming out of the open incisions? Something easy for God!

So understand that you may not understand everything, nonetheless, respect what you may not know as long as it does not harm you. What do you have to lose? In so keeping, dedicate the healing to the Creator of All Things and give thanks and respect to the process by honoring the process and the prescribed manners of the process.

Charity given in any direction that is dedicated to thank the process of healing and attribute it to Him alone, God Almighty, provides enormous benefit and protection. Say, "on behalf of the benefit I received and am not worthy of, I give to this homeless person." Whatever you are able to afford, a meal, or even a dime. A smile is charity and carries with it great benefit. Money should be given to the healer as a gift to ensure these services are available to others and that the healer, dedicating themselves to help humanity, is properly cared for.

Many patients have come to us for Hijama after spending thousands of dollars on conventional doctors and treatments with no beneficial results. We often spend hours on the phone and in consultation with them to arrive at a better understanding of their particular needs and condition. Many times we feed them both dinner and breakfast. They come for Hijama, sometimes from great distances spending hundreds of dollars to travel to us. Then when they arrive they offer very little in the way of a donation for our services. We are not mentioning this to complain as all rewards come from Allah alone and our reward is best given by Him, but we do feel compelled to mention this reality as it is harming the practice of Hijama and keeping it from being available to others. We are always gracious and thank people for what they have offered, but on the whole the offering is a fraction of what they would have paid to a doctor or health care provider. Then they call us on the phone and say how much better they feel, how much money we saved them from having to go to doctors, and how much they appreciate what we have done. We have done nothing, but without supporting the practitioners offering these services they will disappear. Just as those offering your children Qur'an lessons need to be highly compensated for their efforts, otherwise people will find these services less and less available. If not supporting real Hijama practitioners, the only persons left will be those businessmen and women who are savvy in packaging and marketing their services.

Those who charge large upfront fees are normally frauds with no ijaaza to perform Hijama, people who are turning Hijama into a business. By disrespecting the practitioner who is providing authorized services you permit the frauds to flourish and control the services offered. We all get the leaders, Sheikhs, teachers and practitioners we deserve. If the Ummah (community) of Prophet Muhammad (saws) does not support authentic and authorized practitioners of Hijama then there will be none to blame for the absences of this service than the people themselves.

### Cautions & Dangers

Hijama can be dangerous if not performed properly. Aggressive treatments on several different parts of the body are to be avoided. Treatment performed outside of the optimal odd lunar calendar, last half of the lunar month, on spring and fall days is not recommended except in emergency situations.

When the procedure is performed correctly and follow-up directions observed, there is very little risk involved with Hijama. One out of every twenty-five people may experience some lightheadedness and some may even faint. This is normally the result of not having followed the preliminary restrictions or possibly due to weakness from an oncoming cold or flu. The real danger is falling and hitting your head as we always perform Hijama in the seated position facing a prescribed Qiblah direction. With proper monitoring this danger is greatly minimized. Any signs of dizziness or cold sweats should be reported immediately to the practitioner.

### Massage or Dry Cupping

The popularity of massage cupping has grown in recent years and is now being offered as the latest treatment at many spas and by massage therapists looking to expand their services. As stated above, the main risks associated with cupping are from blood clotting. Massage therapists who draw dead blood cells to the surface of the skin and do not extract the dead blood cells from the body are greatly increasing the chance of blood clotting. While short sessions of cupping that do not cause red marks or bring dead blood cells to the surface may not carry any dangers of blood clotting, the benefits do not outweigh the potential risks and we recommend not utilizing this massage technique. As soon as cups are placed on the skin, dead blood cells start to be drawn from the body to the specific site. Massage alone is sufficient to promote circulation and healing - cupping should be reserved for removing dead blood cells from the body.

## Conclusions in Summary

Websites on cupping are now offering certification utilizing information and methods that are harmful. They are attempting to unionize the industry and profit from establishing cupping as a business venture. Ideally, a Hijama practitioner should be compensated, but as a gift, not a fee. In our society this understanding is almost completely lost, so we are not faulting those who charge for their services, simply advocating the method that brings the best results - physically and spiritually.

Despite our many warnings, the Hijama industry (for lack of a better term) will inevitably go the same way as the rest of the medical industry has proceeded. That medical industry is doing much harm and actually promotes more disease than it cures. When profit becomes the motive over service unto your Lord, the benefits of Hijama as well as all other remedies is greatly diminished.

People are free to choose what practitioners are offering the most accurate information on Hijama. Our recommendation is to be very selective and conservative when allowing someone to perform Hijama. Abide by the rule not to sleep after the procedure, and the only thing you should lose is your money and time if not finding a good practitioner, God willing, not your health.

Many people wishing to start a Hijama practice have contacted us and spent hours on the phone questioning us. We are happy to share information about Hijama with anyone who is interested. Unfortunately, most are interested in making money and ignore the warnings and advice we offer - as we predicted. There is nothing wrong with making money, but not at the expense of providing substandard or incorrect Hijama services. Soon new practitioners will organize and attempt to require a license to practice, making it easier to charge higher amounts for Hijama services - not to protect patients, but to profit more through protectionist measures. Efforts have already been made to do just that. Standards for Hijama should be established not from organizing but from adhering to the age old apprentice (ijazaa) practice of receiving training from an authorized Hijama Master. All attempts to do otherwise are an attempt to destroy Islam. There is no better way to protect the practice of Hijama than the ijaaza system rooted in high moral standards and good character.

This information is being offered here to help keep dubious practitioners from performing incorrect Hijama procedures on patients. By educating people on the correct methods of Hijama we hope to improve Hijama treatments provided by practitioners who will insist on turning Hijama into a cupping business centered service, no matter how many warnings we provide. With the information provided in this book we are hopeful that patients will be able to keep practitioners honest and avoid many problems.

We should all work to keep the practice of Hijama as close to the methods utilized and prescribed by Prophets and Saints as possible. So much religious knowledge is being presented as academic knowledge. The spiritual aspect of religious understanding is being buried in the arguments and debates coming from people who like the following example - claim to know about marriage from reading 100 books on the subject but who have never actually been married or loved. They are foolish people (devils) claiming to know something they know nothing about. If you want to learn about marriage you must go to your heart. When you have further questions you must go to someone who knows, like your grandparents - people with real experience who can provide good advice.

What works best with all healing methods and treatments is a full understanding that all cures come from the Creator. Keeping one's heart clean and focused on the real healer is the first step in becoming a vessel through which healing can flow to your fellow man.

## Acknowledgment

How shall an infant describe a noble king and his weighty responsibilities? How shall a fetus describe that which is outside of its immediate enclosed environment? If able to peer outside, how could it understand or even begin to describe its mother's love and her role in its own development. Imagine also that over the course of the child's life the visible love from the mother is but a mere drop in an ocean of love that is concealed and yet known.

Then too, how shall a foolish student, having traveled only a short distance along the endless spiritual path and blessed to follow one so high and noble, describe what he can hardly understand and what he has never seen nor experienced?

This student, dare he even pretend to be a student, is more likened to a baby, so helpless, always soiling himself and in need of cleaning. How might it be possible to describe the mother's role to the child and the infant's need of the mother, through the eyes of the infant who has never had a mother before?

We must, therefore, confess that while describing our beloved Sheikh and Master, we know almost nothing of who he really is and what responsibilities and functions he performs at the behest of his own teacher and under the guidance of the Noblest of all Mankind, our beloved Master Muhammad (saws) for the pleasure of Almighty God.

Each living thing that absorbs a raindrop's worth of water metabolizes it in its own way. Each living thing expounds and glorifies its Lord in its own unique way. How, then, may the moss reflect on how the rose absorbs and metabolizes the same water and nutrients, then produces such varied shapes, colors, aromas and sizes? Even if we considered ourselves to be on a level of a real saint of God, could we ever really know another persons own unique secrets and gifts?

It is far too difficult to answer the question, who is Sheikh Nazim al-Haqqani or what gifts he possesses or to begin to speak about the tools he has been afforded to accomplish those things which have been written for him to accomplish. The best we can do is to invite the infant to enjoy suckling the milk from its mother; revel in the unique sound of the heartbeat of her nurturing embrace, bask in the love which is given by permission — an order of the Most Merciful, and experience and grow from the care and support she (true Sheikh's) provide.

For what does it matter to a child if, upon being born, its mother is only described and not experienced — never presenting the one to the other? How would the description of its mother ever suffice the baby's need for a real mother?

To begin to know Sheikh Nazim al-Haqqani is to meet him and connect your heart to his heart. Then a glimpse of what is possible may come, followed by endless glimpses of things not yet known until you begin to realize he has been there all along.

It is a fact that, when you are ready, your teacher will come.

We thank God Almighty for having guided us to such a noble one. Our words, actions and thoughts are not sufficient to give thanks for our mother's milk let alone the depths of spiritual enlightenment and nutrition God has provided us through His true ones, the real saints, the pole of creation, the proof of generosity.

Forgive us oh Lord, for being so deficient in conveying that which cannot be conveyed in mere words and letters. Help us to achieve a better understanding of who Sheikh Nazim al-Haqqani is and make us better students in our service unto You, Almighty Lord.

We would be seriously remiss if not paying tribute and asking blessing upon Sheikh Abu Bashar for providing our initial Hijama training, Sheikh Adnan Kabbani, Allah bless his many secrets, said to be the number one Awliya (Saint) of our time, who spent hours upon hours trying to teach us how to sit still and listen (learn). Much blessings and peace upon Sheikh Mehmet whose important position in these times will be made evident very soon, and a special mention and show of allegiance to His Royal Highness, the Caliphate of the Muslim Nation, King Abdullah II of Jordan.

Endless praise and peace be upon our Master Muhammad (saws), his family, and companions.

For the honor of the most honored amongst creation, saydinah Muhammad (saws),

Al-Fatiha(The Opening Verse).

## Appendix I.
## Hadith regarding the Sunnah of Hijama

The following information was taken from sources on the Internet and can therefore not be individually verified as authentic translations or reputable hadith. They are being offered for information purposes only. Hadith scholarship must be provided by someone who understands the totality of information provided by the Prophet (saws) so that the wisdom and total meaning of a particular saying can be applied. Similar to the need to have an ijaaza to practice Hijama, people who are offering or transmitting hadith require an ijaaza. Too many unauthorized practitioners use some of the following hadith to validate their practice rather than validating proper hijama practices with an ijaaza. Readers are therefore encouraged to consult authorized hadith scholars before applying the following knowledge to the practice of Hijama. The strength and validity of the information may or may not be able to be relied upon as sound.

Anas ibn Maalik reported that the Messenger said, "Indeed the best of remedies you have is cupping (Hijama)..." [Saheeh al-Bukhaaree (5371)].

Abu Hurairah reported that the Messenger said, "If there was something excellent to be used as a remedy then it is cupping (Hijama)." [Saheeh Sunan abi Dawud (3857), Saheeh Sunan ibn Maajah (3476)].

Abdullah ibn Abbas reported that the Messenger said, "I did not pass by an angel from the angels on the night journey except that they all said to me: Upon you is cupping (Hijama), O Muhammad." [Saheeh Sunan ibn Maajah (3477)].

In the narration reported by Abdullah ibn Mas'ud the angels said, "Oh Muhammad, order your Ummah (nation) with cupping (Hijama)." [Saheeh Sunan Tirmidhee (3479)].

Anas ibn Maalik reported that the Messenger said, "Whoever wants to perform cupping (Hijama) then let him search for the 17th, 19th and 21st day (of the Islamic, lunar month) and let none of you allow his blood to rage (boil) such that it kills him." [Saheeh Sunan ibn Maajah (3486)].

Anas ibn Maalik reported that the Messenger said, "When the weather becomes extremely hot, seek aid in cupping (Hijama). Do not allow your blood to rage (boil) such that it kills you." [Reported by Hakim in his 'Mustadrak' and he authenticated it and Imam ad-Dhahabi agreed (4/212)].

Jaabir ibn Abdullah reported that the Messenger said, "Indeed in cupping (Hijama) there is a cure." [Saheeh Muslim (5706)].

Ibn Umar reported that the Messenger said, "Cupping (Hijama) on an empty stomach* is best. In it is a cure and a blessing..." [Saheeh Sunan ibn Maajah (3487)].

Abu Hurairah reported that the Messenger said, "Whoever performs cupping (Hijama) on the 17th, 19th or 21st day (of the Islamic, lunar month) then it is a cure for every disease." [Saheeh Sunan abi Dawud (3861)].

Anas ibn Maalik reported that the Messenger said, "Whoever wants to perform cupping (Hijama) then let him search for the 17th, 19th and 21st..." [Saheeh Sunan ibn Maajah (3486)].

Ibn Umar reported that the Messenger said, "Cupping (Hijama) on an empty stomach* is best. In it is a cure and a blessing. It improves the intellect and the memory. So cup yourselves with the blessing of Allah on Thursday. Keep away from cupping (Hijama) on Wednesday, Friday, Saturday and Sunday to be safe. Perform cupping (Hijama) on Monday and Tuesday for it is the day that Allah saved Ayoub from a trial. He was inflicted with the trial on Wednesday. You will not find leprosy except (by being cupped) on Wednesday or Wednesday night." [Saheeh Sunan ibn Maajah (3487)].

Ibn Umar reported that the Messenger said, "Cupping (Hijama) on an empty stomach* is best. It increases the intellect and improves the memory. It improves the memory of the one memorizing. So whoever is going to be cupped then (let it be) on a Thursday in the name of Allah. Keep away from being cupped on a Friday, Saturday and Sunday. Be cupped on a Monday or Tuesday. Do not be cupped on a

Wednesday because it is the day that Ayoub was befallen with a trial. You will not find leprosy except (by being cupped) on Wednesday or Wednesday night." [Saheeh Sunan ibn Maajah (3488)].

Salmat, the servant of the Messenger said, "Whenever someone would complain of a headache to the Messenger of Allah he would advise them to perform cupping (Hijama)." [Saheeh Sunan abi Dawud (3858)].

Ibn al-Qaiyum (may Allah have mercy on him) mentions that the Messenger was cupped on his head when he was afflicted with magic and that it is from the best of cures for this if performed correctly. [Zaad al Ma'aad (4/125-126)].

Abdullah ibn Abbas reported that a Jewish woman gave poisoned meat to the Messenger so he sent her a message saying, "What caused you to do that?" She replied, "If you really are a Prophet then Allah will inform you of it and if you are not then I would save the people from you!" When the Messenger felt pain from it, he performed cupping (Hijama). Once he travelled while in Ihram and felt that pain and hence performed cupping (Hijama). [Ahmed (1/305) the hadeeth is hasan (good chain with all the paths)].

Ibn Umar reported that the Messenger said, "Cupping (Hijama) on an empty stomach* is best. In it is a cure and a blessing. It improves the intellect and the memory..." [Saheeh Sunan ibn Maajah (3487)].

Jaabir ibn Abdullah reported that the Messenger fell from his horse onto the trunk of a palm tree and dislocated his foot. Waki' t said, "Meaning the Messenger was cupped on (his foot) for bruising." [Saheeh Sunan ibn Maajah (2807)].

Abdullah ibn Abbas reported that the Messenger was cupped on his head for a unilateral headache while he was in Ihraam. [Saheeh al-Bukhaaree (5701)].

Abdullah ibn Abbas reported that the Messenger was cupped while he was fasting. [Saheeh al-Bukhaaree (5694)].

Anas ibn Maalik was asked: "Did you dislike cupping for the fasting person?" He said, "No except for the reason of one becoming weak." [Saheeh al-Bukhaaree (1940)].

It is god to note her that being a sunnah of Prophet Muhammad Hijama is therefore blessed and the extracted blood from the body does not invalidate your purification (wudu).

Abu Sa'eed al-Khudhree said, "The Messenger validated cupping for the fasting person." [Saheeh see Irwaa al-Ghaleel (4/74)].

Anas ibn Maalik reported that the Messenger was treated with cupping (Hijama) three times on the two veins at the side of the neck and the base of the neck. [Saheeh Sunan abi Dawud (3860), ibn Maajah (3483)].

Abdullah ibn Abbas reported that the Messenger was cupped on his head. [Saheeh al-Bukhaaree (5699)].

Abdullah ibn 'Umar reported that the Messenger used to cup his head and would call it (the place at the top of the head) "Umm Mugheeth." [Saheehah (753), Saheeh al-Jaami' (4804)].

Jaabir ibn Abdullah reported that the Messenger was treated with cupping (Hijama) on his hip for a pain in that area. [Saheeh Sunan abi Dawud (3863)].

Anas ibn Maalik reported that the Messenger was treated with cupping (Hijama) when he was in Ihram, on the top of his foot, for a pain in that area. [Saheeh Sunan abi Dawud (1836)].

Ibn al-Qayyim (may Allaah have mercy on him) said, "Cupping (Hijama) under the chin is beneficial for pain in the teeth, face and throat, if it is performed in its proper time. It purifies the head and the jaws.

Cupping (Hijama) on the top of the foot is a substitution for the puncturing of the Saphena, which is a large vein in the heel. It is beneficial for treating ulcers that occur on the thighs and calves, the interruption of menses and skin irritation on the testicles.

Cupping (Hijama) at the bottom of the chest is beneficial for the treatment of sores, scabies and mange on the thighs. It helps against gout, hemorrhoids, elephantiasis and itchiness on the back." [Zaad al-Ma'aad, 4/58].

Jaabir ibn Abdullah reported Umm Salama (may Allah be pleased with her) asked permission from the Messenger to be treated with cupping (Hijama). So the Messenger ordered Abu Teeba to cup her. Jaabir ibn Abdullah y said, " I think he said that Abu Teeba is her brother through breastfeeding or a young boy who didn't reach puberty". [Saheeh Muslim (5708), abu Dawud (4102), Saheeh ibn Maajah (3480)].

## Appendix II. Bibliography of Source Material

Breathing: The Master Key to Self-Healing, Andrew Weil M.D. Audio CD 1999.

The Prime Cause and Prevention of Cancer, 1967 Dr. Otto Warburg. Lecture June 30, 1966.

Oxygen Healing Therapies, Nathaniel Altman 1995, 1998.

Journal of Experimental Medicine.

Conscious Breathing, Gay Hendricks, PhD, 1995.

The Breathing Book, Donna Farhi, 1996.

The Breath Connection, Robert Fried, PhD, 1990.

Oxygen Breakthrough, Sheldon Saul Hendler, MD, Ph.D.

The Textbook on Medical Physiology, Dr. Arthur C. Guyton, M.D. And John E. Hall, 1996.

The Power of Breathing, Dr. Sukhraj S. Dillon, 2011.

## Recommended Reading

Natural Medicine, Traditional Sufi Healing Methods, Sheik Nazim Al Haqqani an Naqshbandia, 1997.

Made in the USA
Monee, IL
08 November 2026

67994720R00080